MAKING SENSE OF HEALTH

DR TIM O'DOWD

MAKING SENSE OF HEALTH

The Prevention
Playbook to Safeguard
Your Future Health

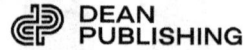

DEAN PUBLISHING

First published in 2025 by Dean Publishing
PO Box 119
Mt. Macedon, Victoria, 3441
Australia
deanpublishing.com

Cataloguing-in-Publication Data
National Library of Australia

Title: Making Sense Of Health
ISBN: 978-0-648758-07-5
Category: Health & Wellbeing

For Jennifer, my Lady in Red.

The scientists, researchers, and investigative
journalists who continue to question…
Volek, Phinney, Noakes, Ioannidis,
Harcombe, Fettke, Taubes, Teicholz,
Kendrick, and previous heroes…
Barker, Cahill, Reaven, Hallberg, Kraft.

CONTENTS

"It is easy to dodge
our responsibilities,
but we cannot dodge
the consequences
of dodging our
responsibilities."

– Sir Josiah Stamp

MAKING SENSE OF HEALTH – WHY?

Eighty percent of the Australian population live with and suffer from chronic diseases.

HOWEVER

The risk of developing a chronic disease can be reduced substantially.

FIRST

Become aware of the factors that promote or degrade health.

THEN

Use *The Prevention Playbook* to *Safeguard Your Future Health.*

There is one sure fact about the human life cycle: death is inevitable. I can safely add that those who are inherently healthy, through genetics, good fortune, or through their own effort, are more likely to have an above average life expectancy. However, over 80 percent of the Australian population live with and suffer from one or more chronic diseases for many years before they die.[1] These chronic disorders don't just happen the day your doctor gives you a diagnosis. There is a long lag time, sometimes as long as 2 or 3 decades, and warning signs that I refer to as Red Flags should ring the alarm bells long before you walk out of the doctor's surgery with an unwelcome diagnosis. Often, however, these health warnings are not considered in the context of the gradual degradation of your overall health. When it comes to chronic disease, the warning signs are always there, and taking action early is likely to prevent disaster later on.

Making sense of the conflicted information about health is a challenge for everyone, doctors included. For the average Australian interested in maintaining or returning to health, confusion can destroy their enthusiasm, or send them on a path doomed to lead to failure. What you read is often a reflection of the author's biases, even if there are reams of 'data' supporting their claims.

Reliable information is knowledge. Knowledge in turn gives you the option to choose your health destiny.

The main goals of *Making Sense of Health* are to present my assessment of the options to enhance and preserve health, to help you understand what might degrade your health, and to make you aware of any external influences.

I focus on your ability to control as much as possible regarding your lifelong health, seeing beyond the recommendations that are failing to achieve reasonable population health, understanding the corporate and institutional contribution to poor health outcomes, disconnecting from the 24-hour news and social media cycles, giving you my translation of the improved medical science that has resulted in exciting successes in achieving good health, and now, hopefully, inspiring you to make goals for your own pursuit of good health.

NAVIGATING THE EVER-SHIFTING LANDSCAPE OF HEALTH AND WELLNESS

My nearly 50-year career as a doctor and specialist was governed by a desire to serve, care for, and respect patients, their relatives, my nursing and medical colleagues, and the myriad of workers who contribute to these goals. It was a privileged position. Newer breakthroughs in scientific understandings, treatments, and technologies demanded a continuous upgrading of my medical education.

I had been a doctor for 13 years when I first became aware of Professor David Barker. His research concerned the origins of a range of chronic diseases. At that stage, I had recently commenced my career as an obstetrician and gynaecologist. I was confident in the knowledge and experience I had amassed from medical school and specialist training. There had been a lot to learn, too much in fact to ever think of questioning the evidence behind it. Academia and its professors were in exalted positions of authority. They had control over my exam results and career promotions. Dissent might invite chastisement.

Twenty-seven years later in 2011, Professor Barker gave the prestigious Sir Richard Doll Lecture in London, where he stated: "Coronary heart disease, type 2 diabetes, breast cancer and many other chronic diseases are unnecessary. Their occurrence is not mandated by genes passed down to us through thousands of years of evolution. Chronic diseases are not the inevitable lot of humankind."[2]

Wow! That was a lightbulb moment in my career. We had believed that with ageing comes health deterioration and the occurrence of various chronic diseases. This is true to a degree. Humans are living a life cycle where functions decline in the last year or two before death. The big concern now, the big change in the mid-2020s, is that the onset of chronic diseases is happening earlier in the life cycle, and their prevalence is increasing at a great rate. These chronic diseases are a concern for the government, the healthcare system, and all Australians. So, what is going wrong with people's health despite all the hype about breakthroughs?

Professor Barker's lecture coincided with my own desires to reduce weight and become physically fitter. And so, I began to sift through all the noise and agendas in the confusing media and scientific literature. I began to grapple with all I had been taught and with the collection of practice guidelines that medical colleges and government health authorities published.

No matter what our roles are in life – parenting, professional, trade – we may have accepted ideas that need remodelling. I recalled the words of Dr David Sackett, the so-called 'father of evidence-based medicine': "Half of what you'll learn in medical school will be shown to be either dead wrong or out of date within five years of graduation; the trouble is that nobody can tell you which half – so the important thing to learn is how to learn on your own."[3]

My unquestioning acceptance of academic health information became infused with critical analysis and a little dose of scepticism. Well-intentioned tenets and dogma in medicine must be continually assessed against the associated outcomes. Clearly, now, despite the tremendous benefits of modern medicine, there is a need for a reassessment. The worsening prevalence of chronic diseases like obesity, type 2 diabetes, and dementia, suggests a re-evaluation of what Australians can do to lower their risks of developing these conditions.

THE CURRENT STATE OF AFFAIRS

The human body is superbly complex, resilient, and adaptable – and in need of your support!

Despite exposure to all sorts of dangers, from threatening situations, injuries, and infections, your body has mechanisms to facilitate rapid responses to these acute upsets, allowing repair and recovery. In other words, most people will have temporary encounters with reduced health, but generally the body has the ability to cope with these, and a return to good health can be expected.

We need to know the factors that support the proper function of the body's internal coping mechanisms. In addition, the superb body is also vulnerable, and so we need to know the factors that degrade its normal coping responses.

The body's ability to adapt can become overwhelmed. Over time, the acute responses to health issues become prolonged, developing into what we refer to as 'chronic diseases' (also referred to as chronic non-communicable diseases). This is the situation for too many Australians who are now living with one or more chronic diseases, diseases that reduce their quality of life, increase their dependency on the healthcare system, and often reduce their life expectancy. A chronic disease is a long-lasting poor health condition with persisting effects, usually for the remainder of the person's life.

The susceptibility to disease has held a fascination for humans for centuries. From philosophers and scientists to many well-meaning enthusiasts, our understanding of the physiology and pathology of the human body has progressed substantially. Yet it remains incomplete. There is a never-ending search for the secret(s) to a healthy life, free from the consequences of disease. Theories abound, research and management rabbit holes are negotiated, and apparent breakthroughs are advertised regularly.

Healthcare practitioners are caring professionals who must rely on researchers continuing to explore the mysteries of health, disease, and wellbeing. Doctors have a difficult job. All patients are individuals with differing presentations, even for the same underlying problems. Their home lives, personal safety, employment, finances, goals, and wishes all play a part. So, the doctor must explore the patient's circumstances before jumping to diagnostic conclusions, investigations, and treatments.

Wonderful advances in technology and blood tests aid diagnosis. Medical knowledge in peer-reviewed journals and guidelines is said to double every 60 days! No doctor can keep up with this. Recommendations are suggested by authoritative institutions, and doctors feel they are obliged to act on these. However, many healthcare guidelines, although well-intentioned when introduced, were based on poor supporting evidence. Additionally, guidelines have assumed an elevated role, virtually unchallengeable, overriding the healthcare practitioner's wisdom gained from knowledge and experience. The guidelines may even challenge the patient's goals and wishes. Also, some exciting new knowledge takes years to be accepted and put into practice – for example, the remissions possible in type 2 diabetics when they make low-carb nutritional changes.

Much of the practice of medicine has been geared at *diagnosis and treatment* of diseases. Developments geared at diagnosis and treatment will continue to assist doctors and other healthcare specialists to improve the quality of life for those of us who become unwell. Patients present for help because of some concerning symptoms. These may be due to pathology that has been evolving for years and presumably could have been avoided. Damage to functions or organs may have become virtually irreversible. In this situation, the doctor's options are limited to medications or surgery. So, in thinking back to Professor Barker's quote, I believe we should plan to help our bodies function, by maintaining cellular and whole-body health, thereby reducing the risk of developing chronic diseases and **preventing** them in the first place.

To suggest that it is possible to prevent chronic diseases is somewhat presumptive on my part. Yet, I am not alone in advocating for preventative action. My thoughts about chronic disease prevention are actually advocated by the WHO (World Health Organization), our own Australian Government, and many eminent organisations. The recent outstanding successes in the nutrition management of type 2 diabetes have opened the door to all who care for their future health to undertake the steps that are known to be fundamental requirements of our human bodies and to limit those factors that sabotage health.[4] Your health is, to a great degree, fashioned by your own efforts. No, there is no guarantee, but there is an option – prevention.

MY APPROACH TO MAKING SENSE OF HEALTH

Our human body is a superbly complex system, ranging from the visible whole to tiny, microscopic cells and their thousands of internal organelles. Somewhat akin to society where there are layers of hierarchy, from babies to leaders, all busily carrying out their roles, every little part of the body contributes to its whole functionality.

Humans have forever sought to understand how this elaborate and intricate system works. While we have learnt so much, the deeper that scientists probe, the greater the complexity and confusion.

I am reminded of Aristotle's observations that the whole is greater than the sum of its parts and the behaviour of complex systems, like the human organism, cannot be explained from an analysis of its individual components.

And so it is with health! Despite the depth of understanding regarding the body, health, and disease, we are facing more cancer, diabetes, dementia, and mental health problems than in previous eras.

Despite my years as a doctor, keeping up to date with medical matters, I, too, became confused when conflicting information challenged long-held 'truths'. How was I to make sense of health? Had progress in health sciences become lost in the nitty-gritty, trying to reveal the merits or harm of some unpronounceable chemical? Should everyone take a multi-pill?

It was time to reassess my understanding of health, leave

behind arguments like whether eggs are good or bad for health, and return to two basic principles:

1. Understand the essential factors the human body requires to function optimally, thereby promoting, maintaining, or restoring health.
2. Understand the factors that degrade health.

Making Sense of Health is my assessment of the confused and conflicted literature on health. I make a plea that you support your body with its essential requirements, and I strongly suggest that you become aware of the players who have academic, political, or financial interests in the business of health.

STUDY THE PLAYBOOK, MASTER THE GAME

Health (and its nemesis, disease) is a vast subject. It involves a combination of brilliant scientific endeavours and enormous reams of research articles, but it is plagued with confusion, myths, and missed opportunities. It is very difficult to tease out information that will reliably benefit all Australians.

Many people are too busy to critically explore and make sense of what they should do to optimise their long-term health. Unfortunately, diabetes, and the chronic diseases of heart, brain, kidneys, and cancers, develop gradually over the years, more or less 'under the radar', until finally the doctor makes an official diagnosis.

Making Sense of Health is my analysis of problems, debates, and opportunities relating to the health of Australians like you, what your body requires to function in a healthy fashion, and what exposes it to increased risks of degrading function, a chronic disease diagnosis, and the subsequent consequences. When you become fully aware of what supports and what threatens your precious body, you can develop a playbook for how best to safeguard your future health.

Making sense of health is a lot like climbing a mountain. The first step is to prepare for your ascent by learning the basics and understanding the journey ahead. The next step is to climb the mountain of information, avoiding hazards (misinformation) along the way. The final step is to reach the summit, where you can see everything clearly and are ready to put your new-found knowledge into action. Your journey to safeguard your future health starts now.

PREVENTION PLAYBOOK
CHAPTER SUMMARY

There is ample but conflicting health information. Reliable information is knowledge. Understand why health knowledge gives you the opportunity to safeguard your health destiny.

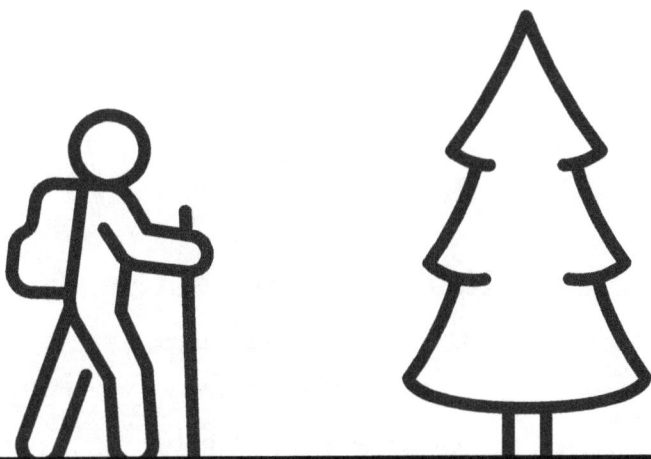

Part 1

BEGIN THE JOURNEY
(EXPLORATION OF HEALTH)

Health is a concept –
difficult to define,
something we
desire, especially
when we lose it.

Chapter 1

HEALTH – AN ENIGMA THAT DEFIES DEFINITION

When you or I make 'health' a goal, it would seem wise to understand what we mean by the word.

Let's start with a few questions.

- What does the word 'health' mean to you?
- Is it an all-embracing term identified with good health, failing health, poor health, bad health?
- Is 'health' the opposite end of the spectrum from 'disease'?
- Is it a theoretical level of perfection, a holy grail, the best you?

- Is it a state of the body when we are in between pesky viral illnesses?
- Is health synonymous with being physically fit?
- Can you be healthy if you have a disability?
- Can you truly be healthy in mind and body if you were abused as a child, if you are living in an abusive relationship, or if you are trying to survive in the terrible humanitarian crisis of a war?

But first, a few interesting phrases you may have heard:

a. Life expectancy. The expected number of living years between birth and death. In Australia, the figure is lower for males, 81 years, and higher for females, 85 years.[1]

b. Life span. This term is often used and misused. It actually means the greatest age reached by humans – currently about 120 years. Sometimes it is used instead of life expectancy.

c. Health span. The number of years someone lives healthy and free of chronic disease, retaining adequate movement and cognition. It is concerning that many people in Australia have one or more chronic diseases for a decade before their eventual death, which often occurs prematurely, before age 75.

d. Soul span. Cardiologist Dr Paddy Barrett uses this term, suggesting the duration of purpose and fulfilment in life.

Surprisingly, 'health' has many interpretations. You may have your personal definition, and there are numerous expert articles that attempt to create a definition appropriate for our times. In addition, definitions of health depend on whether you are a researcher exploring community determinants of disease, or a government policymaker needing to consider health goals and disease prevention for the country while also considering budgetary limitations.

Prior to 1948, 'health' was determined in terms of physical health, that is, the presence or absence of disease. Most deaths back then were due to infections, heart attacks, strokes, cancers, and injuries. Then in 1948, the WHO, through its first director general, Canadian psychiatrist Dr Brock Chisholm, published a definition that dominates journalistic and medical articles even to this day. It states that: "Health is a state of complete physical, mental and social well-being and not merely the absence of disease or infirmity."[2]

Using the WHO definition implies that any functional disability could be considered poor health. In addition, the definition excludes most of us because we know from national and global statistics that chronic diseases are common and trending upwards. In other words, most people are not healthy!

Many academics have challenged the WHO definition and offered alternatives. Should you alone, or some appointed person, a doctor for example, decide that you have "complete physical, mental, and social well-being"? If complete also means complete wellbeing for the long-term, most people could not claim to be healthy, as we all have our sick days. In addition, the phrase "not merely the absence of disease" begs the question of by who and what means is it determined whether a disease is absent? Does this involve the absence of certain symptoms and signs at a doctor's examination, or is it determined through simple, or indeed complex, blood tests, X-rays, or other testing? Should everyone have PET or MRI scans?

A favoured definition quoted by many writers is: "Health is a state of balance, an equilibrium that an individual has established within himself and between himself and his social and physical environment."[3]

This suggests that a disease or impairment doesn't necessarily negate a person's feeling that they are adequately healthy – that is, that health is *a personal entity* and may be regarded as having different levels. It may be that the important factor is how the individual in good or poor health, with or without a disease, feels about themselves and how they cope and carry on with their lives.

Even the experts are struggling to give an all-encompassing definition of health.

One could regard health as a broad term reflecting the general condition of the body and mind, implying anything between the positive, 'good' health, and the negative, 'poor' health.

Even though a precise definition is difficult for all to agree on, we probably agree that health is *desirable* yet *variable*, an *expectation* yet *not guaranteed*, a matter of strongly held *opinions* and *confusion*. During our journey from birth, it is desirable to remain in good health for as long as possible and reduce the chance of subclinical and diagnosed states of poor health and their consequences. Good health is like an investment, a resource to help us adapt and cope with the twists and turns of modern living.

There is an element of luck determining where you are on the spectrum between the extremes of good and poor health. So much depends on where you were born, your genetics, your social, economic, political, and physical environment, and the clinical care available. In all countries, there are health and healthcare inequities. Those at the top of the socio-economic ladder living in the larger cities experience fewer of the chronic illnesses compared to those at the lower end and in the distant rural areas.

Recently, I asked my friend Tina what she thought about the word 'health'. Immediately, she replied that she believed that 'health' was *uncertain*! Her wife Jo, slim, fit, and 'healthy', careful about what she eats, was recovering from surgery to fix a bleeding blood vessel in her brain. No prior medical problems. No trauma. Perfectly well one minute, but then the internal bleeding in her brain caused pressure on the speech area. She began to slur her sentences and was finding it difficult to communicate. She was developing a stroke at age 35! Jo's brain abnormality, called an arteriovenous malformation, was probably present from birth but had never previously caused a problem.

For Tina and Jo, 'health' is *precious* and *uncertain*, and *not completely under our control*. Something you think about only when it goes wrong.

There are known *drivers of good health*. These are activities that are associated with supporting your body's essential requirements, factors that are necessary to fuel, mobilise, and rest it to allow it to function at its best. In that way, it can function as it was designed, to exist, to survive, and to heal when required.

There are also many recognised factors and behaviours associated with poor health, which contribute to a dependence on family and the healthcare system to assist with day-to-day living. I will refer to these as *drivers of poor health*.

PREVENTION PLAYBOOK
CHAPTER SUMMARY

———————

Health is a concept – difficult to define, something we desire, especially when we lose it, desirable yet variable, an expectation yet not guaranteed, a matter of strongly held opinions and confusion.

Chapter 2

EXPECTATION OF HEALTH, REALITY OF DISEASE

When in life's journey do you become aware of health, disease, and mortality?

It may be when you or a family member is given a disease diagnosis. Maybe it is when your child is diagnosed with emotional or mental health problems, like anxiety or attention deficit disorder. Or possibly when you hit 40 and the residual fitness of youth has reduced so much that you get puffed kicking a ball with one of your children. Quite often, it takes some shock for most of us to become interested in our mortality and wellbeing, and only then, at this late stage, when we have possibly lost it, does the whole issue of health become a concern – and you won't be alone. Annual national statistics sourced from the Australian Bureau of Statistics and the Australian Institute of Health and Welfare show that chronic diseases are becoming more prevalent, and it is of grave concern that they are occurring at younger ages.[1]

All animals and plants have a life cycle and will eventually die. In the case of humans, there are changes that happen in old age like joint and muscle stiffness, and certainly various organ functions become jaded. The immune system is less capable than in younger days, and an older person becomes more vulnerable to infections and injury. But aging should not automatically result in the development of chronic diseases.

DISEASE PREVENTION – THE KEY IS COMMITMENT

As we shall soon discover, every human body is extraordinarily complex. It is a self-organising system, capable of self-maintenance when fed and watered, and capable of self-healing when confronted with the occasional accident or illness. It is adaptable, responsive to attacks by microorganisms, and able to repair from injury and surgical operations. Its destiny is to function as a unique system, capable of growth, development, reproduction, and, alas, eventually death. It is not unreasonable to expect long-term health. Modern medicine may assist with newer medications, but I believe the expectation of lifelong health must be accompanied by taking personal responsibility, that is, a commitment to prevention of disease.

THE REALITY OF DISEASE

Of course, there are exceptions to the concept of perfect health from birth. As a medical doctor and obstetrician, I was fully aware of those exceptions. Genetic mishaps during pregnancy, childhood and teenage infections and cancers, and unexplained illnesses are significant events requiring intense medical assistance.

However, as I have inferred already, chronic diseases have become a major health burden in Australia and most other countries. Type 2 diabetes, coronary heart disease, major cognitive decline, fatty liver disease, certain cancers, obesity, and other conditions are to a large extent caused by factors related to our lifestyles and should be considered unnecessary.

Even though medical and pharmaceutical approaches to these chronic diseases have had some success at an individual level, the tsunami of new cases, and in younger age groups, seems endless. The present medical approach must be expanded to understand and promote preventative care by the profession itself but also by individuals.

WHY IS THERE SO MUCH DISEASE?

Life, relationships, behaviour, and social, environmental, economic, and political factors exert threats that may overcome the body's normal processes, resulting in dysfunctions of metabolism, the immune system, and the stress response system, which singly or combined lead to one or more chronic diseases.

Factors in our lives create a degree of chronic low-level stress, which causes metabolic disruption due to elevated stress hormones, adrenaline, and cortisol. Sensationalised headlines in the news outlets are common. Everything seems to be a crisis, a catastrophe, or 'unprecedented'. It seems like news outlets are preying on human emotions and creating fear. In the 24-hour news cycle – newspapers, magazines, social media – you are bombarded with breaking stories of environmental disasters, extreme weather events and the negative effects of climate change, devastating wars, forced displacement, fears of further pandemics, as well as escalating costs of living and homelessness.

It is easy to understand that some people feel a loss of control, a fear for the future. It is not a surprise that the continuous portrayal of devastating calamities – no matter how far away – creates a personal response of overwhelming emotion and sympathy as if you are personally involved. The resulting anxiety and stress can impact your wellbeing, your health.

Under the circumstances, it is also easy to understand that you can become distracted from taking personal responsibility for your individual health and wellbeing. It may be beneficial to defocus from the problems of the world and instead focus on the positive outcome you can gain from addressing your own personal health.

SORTING THROUGH THE PILE OF CONFLICTING HEALTH ADVICE

You scour the papers, magazines, podcasts, or the internet for answers but end up with contradictory advice and confusion. The reality of the healthcare industry is that not all advice is accurate, not all 'healthy' foods are healthy even if they carry a high Health Star Rating, and not all healthcare is free from commercial opportunism. It may be difficult to believe that some players in the health industry have ideologically driven agendas that can have negative impacts on your health. Curiously, nutrition guidelines are firmly adhered to by authoritative organisations who, for one reason or another, refuse to accept that the evidence has turned in a different direction.

Of course, if you are confused, or have some worrying or vague symptoms, you can go to a doctor for advice.

Thank goodness for doctors and other healthcare practitioners! What would you do without pathology and diagnostic facilities, hospitals, community support systems, and aged-care facilities? We all need them, whether for health advice, a virus or bacterial illness, chest pain, pregnancy care, trauma management, cancer treatment and survivorship support, and, of course, aged-care support.

CHRONIC DISEASE IN AUSTRALIA

Chronic Diseases Among Australians

Obesity	Hypertension
Mental and behavioural conditions	Anxiety and depression
Arthritis and back problems	Chronic kidney disease
Heart disease (coronary artery disease)	Several cancers (often related to obesity)
Stroke	Fatty liver disease (non-alcoholic/ metabolic dysfunction associated)
Dementia (especially Alzheimer's dementia)	
Type 2 diabetes	Polycystic ovarian syndrome (PCOS)

Unfortunately, there are more Australians living with, and suffering from, chronic illnesses than ever before. As a result, many Australians live 10 years in poor health prior to death. Statistics show us they have worsening mobility and greater dependence on others. In Australia, 80 percent of people over the age of 65 have at least one chronic illness, and 28 percent have three or more and are required to take five or more different medications every day for the remainder of their lives.[2] Side effects from prescribed medications are leading causes of hospital admissions and even death.

Too many people are living with mental and emotional conditions, dementia, obesity, mobility restrictions, diabetes, heart disease, and cancer. Too many people are prescribed too much long-term medication. Too many become dependent on the healthcare industry.

By the time the diagnosis of a chronic disease is made, damage will have already occurred. However, there are several warning signs, '**Red Flags**', that indicate that your body's functions are becoming compromised. These Red Flags predict future poor health outcomes like type 2 diabetes many years before the diagnosis is eventually made. **Early screening for metabolic health could prove to be a breakthrough in reducing the overall burden of chronic diseases in Australia**. The presence of a Red Flag condition will allow you to take preventative action early to help your body's internal networks return to normal function. This is preventative care.

WHERE IS THE PROBLEM?

Where does the problem lie? Is it a problem that doctors are consulted too late to change the course of a disease after it has become established and then diagnosed, when damage is already done? In this regard, medical care is mostly a form of remediation. Medical breakthroughs and dedicated health practitioners are invaluable contributors to the management of established diseases. Yet, despite healthcare budgets that are in the billions and trillions of dollars in Western countries, despite many claims that newer medications will give better outcomes, the fact is that chronic diseases are becoming more prevalent year after year, and life expectancy in the US and Great Britain is reducing and has plateaued in Australia.

THE POWER OF PREVENTION

The potential long-term significance of problems that I refer to as Red Flags (discussed in depth in chapter seven) are often ignored or treated with a pill, sometimes a recommendation to lose weight, but rarely with acknowledgement that they are warnings that radical change in lifestyle habits, such as dietary adjustment, is needed to prevent further progression to chronic disease. This preventative approach could radically reduce subsequent chronic disease becoming established in certain people.

Can we do more, earlier, to prevent the ongoing development of chronic diseases instead of waiting until a diagnosis is finally made? Certainly, this is the opinion stated in the Australian

Government's National Preventive Health Strategy 2021–2030, in which they encourage the need for a more preventative approach to healthcare. In this report, the usual suspects and solutions are discussed: reduce smoking (also vaping), reduce alcohol, improve nutrition, increase participation in physical activities, reduce stress, get early cancer screening. But apart from the usual discussion about good nutrition (more fruits and vegetables), **there is no suggestion to get early metabolic health screening!**

It is estimated that 40 percent of the chronic diseases could be prevented through a reduction in modifiable risk factors, in other words, prevention. At a national level, the proposals will take years to come to fruition, and the authors of the strategy document expect only modest improvements in outcomes.[3]

MORE SCIENCE – MORE HOPE

Help and hope are coming from a rumbling revolution happening in the medical science world. There is a clearer understanding of the drivers of good health and, similarly, the drivers of chronic diseases. Historically, drivers and determinants of diseases included the germ theory, the genetic theory. Now we have entered the 'metabolic theory of disease' era.

To exist, the body relies on efficient production of energy through the work of mitochondria and metabolism. Deterioration in those processes causes metabolic dysfunction. Every cell can be affected, or only the cells in one organ or tissue may be compromised. This makes metabolic dysfunction the supreme troublemaker, even though there may be other factors causing some diseases in some people. Obesity, for example, is a result of metabolic dysfunction, and it is associated with the whole range of chronic diseases. Type 2 diabetes, some cancers, many mental health problems, and some neurodegenerative diseases like Alzheimer's dementia have metabolic origins.

Unfortunately, some health events will occur despite your greatest efforts. However, I firmly believe that you (and your loved ones) can take steps throughout life to lower the risk of developing a chronic disease. It's not complicated. Mostly, it involves understanding how to take advantage of the knowledge and research that I will discuss as we progress through the book. Become aware of what nurtures your body but also of what can destroy it.

Once you develop greater health awareness, you will know how to keep your body's functions in optimal condition, and, as a result, your body will reward you with the longest possible health span.

More complicated than your computer, your human body is awesome and will transport you throughout a long and rewarding healthy life, if you understand it more — and love it and care for it!

PREVENTION PLAYBOOK
CHAPTER SUMMARY

It is not unreasonable to expect long-term
health. Yet long-term chronic diseases are all
too common. Modern medicine may assist
with newer tests and medications, but I believe
the expectation of lifelong health must be
accompanied by taking personal responsibility,
that is, making a commitment to prevention.

"The human body is
superbly complex,
resilient yet vulnerable,
intelligent yet naive,
loved yet abused,
and desperately in
need of repair."

– Tim O'Dowd

Chapter 3

THE INCOMPARABLE HUMAN BODY

Healing secret – you become a new you every 100 days!

Your body should be regarded as a temple – awesome and beautiful. It is a complex, resilient, resourceful organism capable of growth, reproduction, self-repair, and so much more. Even when we are neglectful with our lifestyle choices, it can continue to sustain its existence by continual adaptation, and so much happens beneath the exterior without our conscious awareness. Isn't that extraordinary?

Your body is so much more than a machine with a brain. There are the anatomical structures that everyone is familiar with. The brain and nervous system connecting with every cell in every organ, the pumping heart, the breathing lungs, the digesting gut, the versatile liver, the amazing circulation that visits every cell in the body, kidneys, reproductive organs, and the muscles and bones. And let's not forget the special senses of seeing, hearing, smelling, tasting, and touching that we use to help us interpret our environment.

All the systems in your body's structure, the 37 trillion cells, the organs, the gut, the circulatory system composed of 100,000 kilometres of blood vessels, the nervous, endocrine, and immune systems, all have extensive patterns of connections that are continuously active and interactive.

Then there are processes that involve chemicals, hormones, neurotransmitters, enzymes, and other molecules that maintain the relationships between the structures and facilitate the patterns of instant connection.

Also, there is the mysterious faculty called cognition, which includes all the features of the human mind, like consciousness, the process of knowing, perception, emotion, and action. The scientific understanding of the human mind continues to evolve. Is it a process or a system or both? It is, at the present time, best considered not as a thing or structure, but as processes occurring in the network of neurons and synapses of the central nervous system.

Each human starts out as one solitary cell (embryo) created when the male sperm fertilises the female egg, and by the time of birth there are trillions of cells. An egg is the largest human cell. Sperm, the smallest cells in the body, are 10,000 times smaller than an egg. During IVF (in-vitro fertilisation) procedures, we get the opportunity to see an embryo with the human eye, somewhat like a grain of dust.

Each cell in the body acts like an independent universe carrying out internal functions so it can exist, grow, create energy, maintain and repair its DNA, while also contributing to its specialised external role as part of the brain, the heart, or other tissues or organs. Even though we acknowledge the importance of the nucleus, with its vital DNA, most of the cell's activities are dependent on the healthy functioning of tiny structures called mitochondria.

Cells are continuously active, synthesising and dissolving structures and eliminating waste. These major housekeeping duties include surveillance of all threats from within and from outside the body. There is a never-ending cycle of cell replacement in your skin, organs, tissues, and body fluids. Of the body's 37 trillion cells, 1 percent are replaced daily, suggesting a 'new you' every 100 days. Some cells turn over quickly, for example, the cells lining your gut. Other cells in muscle and fat can last for 15 years. Cells in the heart, eyes, and brain can last a lifetime.[1]

Extraordinary, right? Most of these activities of the body happen under the radar, without your conscious awareness.

But you can consciously influence their proper functioning. You see, despite your body being a self-organising, self-maintaining, and self-renewing entity, it needs your assistance to exist. All functions depend on energy. Every enzyme reaction, every heartbeat, every thought, every movement, requires energy. That energy is produced in mitochondria from the food and drink we consume.

MITOCHONDRIA – THE POWERHOUSE OF THE CELL

The food we eat contains energy and nutrients that are made available to our bodies through the process of metabolism. Every second of human life depends on the ability of the body's 37 trillion cells to convert food energy into its own usable form of energy called ATP (adenosine triphosphate). Every chemical and physical activity is completely dependent on an uninterrupted supply of ATP energy every day. Most of this onerous task is carried out inside each cell in hundreds or thousands of tiny organelles called *mitochondria*.

The process of creating ATP can never stop because it must maintain basic functions like breathing, heartbeat, and digestion, even when you sleep. Also, the brain is very active during sleep, especially during the phase of rapid eye movement, when you are processing memories and dreaming. The production of ATP is lower during sleeping hours, but when you are active, exercising, or put under stress, it must be ramped up, sometimes suddenly.

The availability of ATP allows each cell to make its own proteins, lipids, and other chemicals to make the human body as we know it, with all its inherent properties.

When the process of producing energy from food is perfect, cells use other essential food nutrients to facilitate growth, repair, and reproduction, year after year, until the human life cycle comes to a natural end.

One mitochondrion is tiny. To give you an idea, the width of the nail on your index finger is about 1 cm. Ten thousand to fifty thousand mitochondria would occupy that same width! And there are hundreds to thousands of mitochondria in one cell. They duplicate themselves when more are needed. Each properly functioning mitochondria should be 100 percent efficient at its job. However, in dysfunctional metabolic states, their efficiency is compromised. Their function is dependent on the quality of food molecules and is interfered with by toxins like alcohol, pollutants, chemicals and hormones related to systemic chronic stress and chronic inflammation, as well as excess insulin. When a mitochondrion becomes old or inefficient, it undergoes mitophagy, a process of destruction. Their numbers in a cell can be increased with exercise.

In addition to producing life-sustaining energy, mitochondria have other important roles in human existence. These roles include the production of heat, initiation of inflammation, influencing which sections of our DNA are turned on or off (the process of epigenetics), and the production of hormones like cortisol, oestrogen, and testosterone. During the process of producing ATP, reactive oxygen molecules (free radicals) and antioxidants are also produced. These by-products are usually in balance with each other. When they are out of balance, a state called oxidative stress occurs, and inflammation follows.

Additionally, mitochondria are responsible for housekeeping duties and quality control within each cell. Moreover, mitochondria are geared to self-destruct under some circumstances (mitophagy), as well as dispose of old or defective cells (autophagy). In the brain, toxins produced during the day, for example, beta-amyloid (which is thought to play a major role in Alzheimer's dementia), are disposed of.

As a matter of interest, the well-known poison arsenic has its deadly impact by interfering with ATP production in mitochondria, thereby depleting the cells of energy to function, resulting in death.

Each mitochondrion serves the cell; the cell serves the organ or tissue it has specialised in; the organ serves the body. *The relative health of our mitochondria determines not only whether the body is healthy or not, but whether we exist or not.*

METABOLISM – THE KEY SYSTEM THAT DETERMINES HEALTH

Metabolism refers to the essential, intricate, continuously active body system and process of turning food into:

1. Energy (in mitochondria)
2. Nutrients, that is, the essential molecules required to build, repair, and maintain all the cells, systems, and processes required for the body to function

Metabolism starts with food digestion in the gut. The stomach is a human food mixer, changing food to a fluid consistency. As food moves into the small bowel, enzymes and bile break it down into its basic metabolites – glucose, lipids (fatty acids), amino acids, as well as vitamins and minerals – which can then be absorbed into the blood and lymphatic circulation. Energy contained in glucose and lipids is transformed into the body's own form of energy, ATP. The remaining metabolites (amino acids and lipids, vitamins and micronutrients) are used to build and maintain the body. The body is made from food!

The liver plays an important role in the body (removing toxins, processing food nutrients, and regulating the metabolic process), as does the pancreas (production of enzymes to aid in food digestion and the production of hormones, particularly insulin and glucagon, which are involved in the regulation of blood sugar).

Along with the gastrointestinal tract, the blood circulatory system, with its tireless pump, the heart, distributes metabolites to every cell, where, along with oxygen, they are transformed into water, carbon dioxide, and ATP. The pulmonary system allows us to breathe in oxygen and discard carbon dioxide as we breathe out. Our lungs have an intimate relationship with blood vessels that transport these gases to and from each cell.

A healthy body is the result of normal metabolism, that is, normal metabolic function. However, problems in the processes of metabolism, referred to as metabolic dysfunction, result in problems of health, including excessive weight gain and obesity, high blood pressure, type 2 diabetes, cancer, Alzheimer's dementia, and so on. This is why I say...

To control health, you must control metabolism.

The entire body, each cell, every organ, the muscles, nervous system, the brain, and mind can function only in the presence of energy, combined with the quality of nutrients that we derive from the food we consume. When we support the body with its essential nutrient requirements, and control the factors that compromise normal metabolism, good health should be expected.

METABOLIC DYSFUNCTION (WHEN NORMAL METABOLISM IS OVERWHELMED)

Alas, mitochondrial and metabolic function are vulnerable to personal and external factors that can overwhelm the body's resilience, resulting in poor health and, for some, a shortened life cycle. The consequences of metabolic dysfunction can take years to be recognised as a formal disease diagnosis. However, there are early warning signs, or Red Flags (for example, weight gain, high blood pressure, erectile dysfunction, gestational diabetes, and so on). Recognition of Red Flags provides the opportunity to correct metabolic function and prevent longer-term deterioration.

Our metabolic processes adapted to nature's available (real) foods over thousands of years, but we are now substantially compromising metabolic health through modern foods.

According to a 2023 report on the global burden of disease, diseases related to metabolic dysfunction have shown a significant increase since 2000.[2] Many researchers are calling for an urgent need to identify and implement interventions. In other words, they are identifying the need for prevention.

Since dietary recommendations encouraged businesses to create low-fat, higher-carbohydrate foods, we have damaged the metabolic process. We have changed many food options from recognisable vegetables and fruits, direct from the farm, to ultra-processed packaged 'food' from factories that require nutritional information and ingredient lists, including a list of added man-made chemicals. You can barely read the names of the many added chemicals. Nobody truly understands what role they may have in protecting or damaging your health. Some of these factory foods have endorsements from government-backed organisations that give them inappropriate star ratings, which encourages us to buy them because 'experts' say they qualify as food.

It is unlikely that most chemically altered factory versions of food can satisfy the body's essential nutritional needs. Ultra-processed foods (UPFs) have been shown to be less satiating, creating the need for top-up snacks, which leads to overconsumption. There is also the suggestion that UPFs are addictive, possibly because of the palatability and mouthfeel that comes from salt, sugar, and processed fats. Excess food intake that is not required for immediate use by the body is converted to storage forms like fat. There are numerous studies associating UPFs with a range of metabolically related diseases, including obesity and diabetes. Subsequently, we rely on pharmaceutical chemicals to correct the metabolic problems that the processed food contributes to in the first place.

So, why do we eat UPFs if they sabotage health? In short, the answer is that they are often hyperpalatable, cheap, available everywhere, and convenient for busy families and workers. They also occupy large areas in supermarkets, convenience stores, petrol stations, hospital corridors, and school canteens. Temptation!

HOMEOSTASIS – A KEY PROCESS OF HEALTH SELF-REGULATION

**Homeostasis is a process of self-regulation
to maintain a stable internal environment
within each cell and the body in general.**

There are millions of activities, chemical reactions, and electrical impulses happening every nanosecond. Your body has mechanisms to keep all its systems in a dynamic balance. To maintain balance, there are numerous positive and negative feedback loops between hormones, chemicals, and neurotransmitters that keep these within tolerance levels.

For example, when you eat or drink a sugary food, the level of blood glucose in the circulation may spike quite high. Prolonged high glucose levels in the blood (hyperglycaemia) damage blood vessels throughout the body. To prevent prolonged hyperglycaemia, the pancreas responds by secreting the hormone insulin, which facilitates the entry of glucose into cells, thereby bringing down the glucose level in the circulation into the normal range. If the process is too aggressive and blood glucose levels become too low, another hormone called glucagon stimulates the immediate production of glucose in the liver to bring the blood level back to the accepted normal range.

Similarly, if the body is invaded by a virus, the immune system is activated, and the body allows changes in homeostasis to facilitate the inflammatory response until the virus is neutralised.

When you go to hospital, your vital signs are measured. These reflect the process of homeostasis. Blood pressure, temperature, heart rate (pulse), respiration rate, and a measure of the body's oxygen are usually monitored. In addition, a blood test will check many minerals (such as sodium, potassium, bicarbonate) and molecules (such as haemoglobin, glucose, liver enzymes, cholesterol) to determine if they are within accepted normal range. When there is metabolic or immune system dysfunction, there will be evidence of disrupted homeostasis recognised in the vital signs and blood tests.

On a blood test report, your levels will hopefully be within an accepted normal range. If you are tired, your test may show that haemoglobin and iron levels are too low. If you have a bacterial or viral infection, the white cell count may be elevated, and the body's defence mechanisms will be activated to bring levels back to their normal range. Sometimes an antiviral or antibiotic will be required. If your doctor suspects you may have developed diabetes (a dysfunction of metabolism), testing blood glucose (sugar) levels will aid the diagnosis. From there, dietary adjustment and medications will be used to bring glucose levels back to the normal range.

IMMUNE SYSTEM – THE BODY'S DEFENDER

The immune system responds to acute problems and is an extraordinary part of the body's self-maintenance processes.

It is a very complex and incompletely understood ability of the body to protect itself from attack. Like other systems, it has evolved to assist survival after trauma (including after operations), infections, and pollutants. It relies on cells and molecules recognising the issue, and its response includes directing all sorts of immune cells to isolate, poison, and devour the assailant, and then record a memory to respond even quicker if there is a repeat attack. Inflammation, when redness, pain, and swelling occur, is a usual accompaniment.

When the combat phase of the process has been successful, other chemicals are produced to restore normality. In other words, the *acute immune-inflammatory response* is a self-limiting process that resolves when the threat has been managed.

The immune system also surveys the normality or abnormality of new cells that the body creates. Every day, cells form that could become a cancer. In the presence of healthy metabolism and homeostasis, the abnormal cells will usually be destroyed.

Unfortunately, many factors during human life interfere with stages of the immune-inflammatory process. This is especially true with the resolution stage, resulting in a state of low-grade, sterile, *systemic (whole body) chronic inflammation*. This dysfunctional inflammatory response remains active and long-term. Thus, it can impact normal cellular function, including energy production, as well as all tissues and organs, thereby contributing to chronic diseases.

STRESS RESPONSE – A NATURAL REACTION

Stress can be both a vital and amazing physiological human body response or a prolonged disruptive pathological process. Acute stress response is a physiological and relatively short reaction to some form of internal or external 'stressor' or challenging situation. The source of the stressors can include illness, response to injury or surgery, work or exam deadlines, sleep deprivation, nutritional deficiencies, and of course an immediate physical threat ('fight or flight'). The response is triggered in the brain and involves hormones and the nervous, immune, and metabolic systems, and it has an immediate effect on homeostasis. The impact of the acute stress response affects the heart, lungs, muscles, brain, bowel, and endocrine glands (hormone-producing organs).

In the next chapter, I will discuss the pathological concerns of chronic stress.

PREVENTION PLAYBOOK
CHAPTER SUMMARY

———————

In the normal healthy physiological state, the processes of metabolism, immune reaction, and stress response work together to maintain homeostasis and normal health.

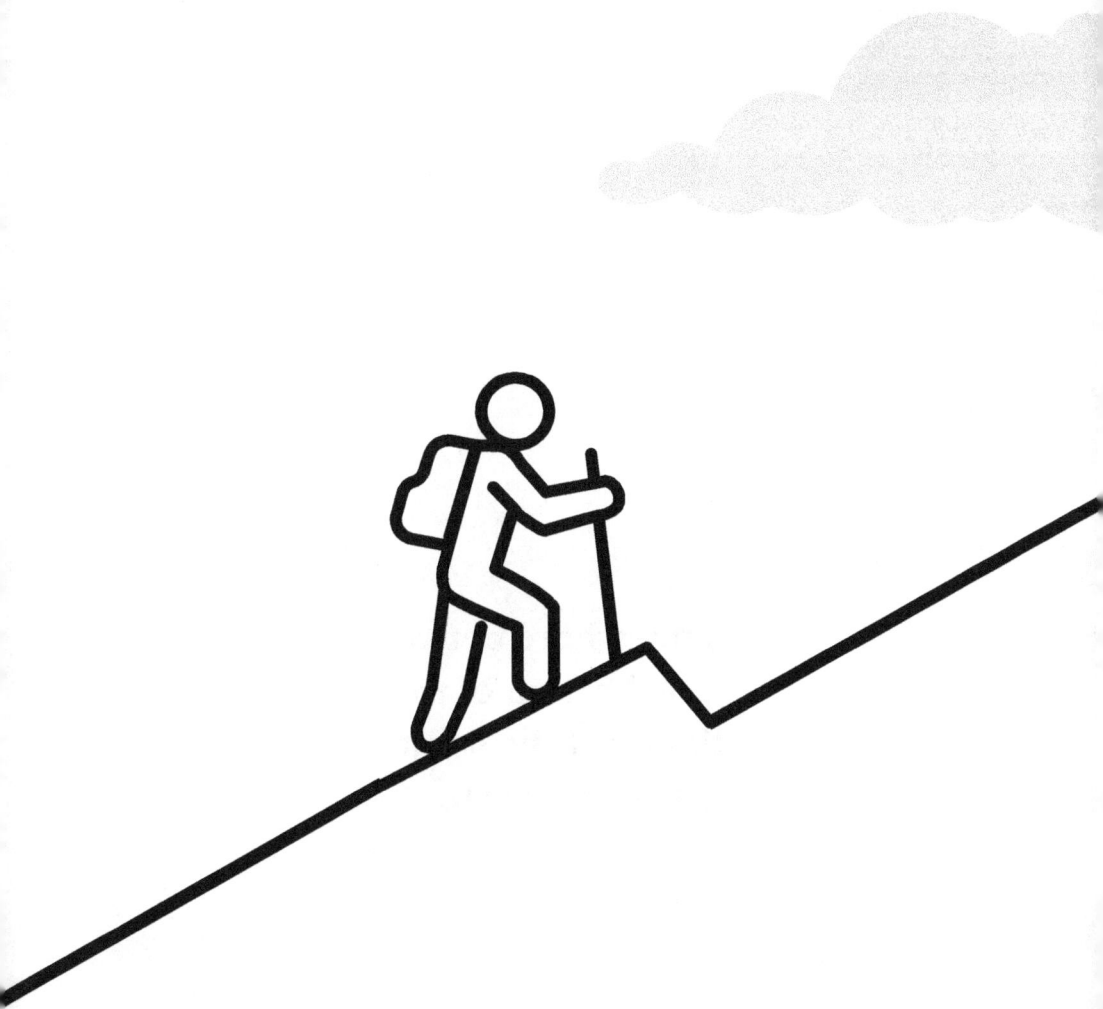

Part 2

CLIMB THE MOUNTAIN
(ACQUIRE KNOWLEDGE)

"Somewhere between
the bottom of the
climb and the summit
is the answer to the
mystery why we climb."

– Greg Child

Chapter 4

THREE COMMON PATHWAYS TO CHRONIC DISEASES

There are several known drivers of chronic diseases, namely genetic, lifestyle, socio-economic, political, and environmental factors. These drivers degrade normal functioning of metabolism, the immune system, or the stress response. When any one of these systems malfunction, they influence one or both of the other functions, as well as homeostasis.

The Big Three Drivers of Disease

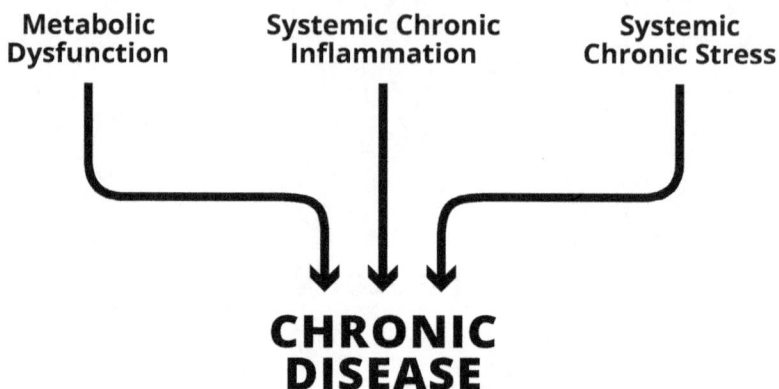

Metabolic   **Systemic Chronic**   **Systemic**
Dysfunction   **Inflammation**   **Chronic Stress**

CHRONIC DISEASE

Thus, metabolic dysfunction, systemic chronic inflammation, and chronic stress are the common pathological pathways that create the various chronic diseases. Because of its importance in creating the energy necessary for life and for every other function that occurs in the human body, metabolic dysfunction must be considered the prime initial contributor or cause of chronic disease.

It has taken me a lifetime in my medical career to unscramble all the knowledge of physiology and pathology that I learnt in medical school and since, and finally I recognise the essential roles that metabolic function and dysfunction play in health. And not only me. It is hitting the medical science world. Diabetes, cancer, neurodegenerative disease, and mental health researchers have discovered the central importance of metabolic function and its relationship to good health of the whole body.

**Most chronic diseases are related to
metabolic dysfunction. Therefore, restoring
normal metabolic function must be the
priority of healthcare and healing.**

METABOLIC DYSFUNCTION

As discussed in previous chapters, **metabolic dysfunction** is a contributor or cause of the development of all the chronic diseases; therefore, attention to metabolic health throughout life could reduce the risk of these disorders occurring in the first place. This knowledge, the significance that there is a modifiable major contributor to chronic diseases, gives everyone the opportunity to improve their metabolic health and reduce or avoid poor health.

There is new compelling evidence that metabolic dysfunction plays a major contributory role in mental health problems. The brain has 85 billion individual neurons (nerve cells), and their normal functioning requires energy. In fact, 20 percent of the body's energy output occurs in the brain, even though it accounts for only 2 percent of body weight. Therefore, it should not be a surprise that any dysfunction in energy availability in the brain from the process of metabolism is likely to contribute or result in mental health disorders. In people who have metabolic dysfunction, adequate glucose enters the brain circulation, but insulin resistance prevents its uptake by cells. Without an adequate energy source, brain cells die. Very-low-carbohydrate or keto diets provide ketones as a perfect fuel replacement.

It is unfortunate that, at this stage, it is uncommon for good dietary advice to be given to individuals living with mental health issues. In the very complex mental health sphere, anxiety, depression, schizophrenia, substance abuse, and bipolar disorder are categorised as separate disorders, even though an individual may have overlapping symptoms and diagnoses. While several non-pharmaceutical therapies are successful for certain behavioural problems, medications are the cornerstone of treatment. Each diagnosis has its own medication treatment regime; however, many psychoactive drugs can be prescribed regardless of the primary diagnosis.

It is exciting that there is a revolution in the understanding of the relationship between mental health and metabolic health. Supporting research is published on a weekly basis concluding that healthier nutrition can not only help the management of established diseases like type 2 diabetes, but may also give us the ability to prevent or manage mental health disorders.

I emphasise the importance of metabolic dysfunction. The US is an example of a country of unparalleled financial wealth, yet it has a shameful health rating. As mentioned, almost 90 percent of its population is considered to have metabolic dysfunction. A similar problem is occurring in countries globally, whether wealthy or not, including Australia.

Even individuals with seemingly perfect health can have an occasional episode of poor health. On that long journey from birth to death, all of us will be exposed to injuries or infections or emotional trauma. It is a normal part of life, and we must accept that our environment or our behaviours will expose us to common colds, sporting injuries, or emotional upsets from social interactions. While you will feel less healthy when you have these issues, they are inclined to be of sudden onset and short-term. Our bodies have the ability to respond to short-term insults, adapt, and compensate using metabolism and the immune and stress systems.

SYSTEMIC CHRONIC INFLAMMATION

Resilience and recovery are built into the systems that comprise the human body. The immune system, with its abundance of chemicals and specialised white blood cells, is unbelievably com-plicated. In short, this system is constantly on call. It acts as a security system to recognise, isolate, and kill abnormal cells in the body (for example, mutated cells that could cause cancer) or intruders (like bacteria, viruses, or fungi) introduced from outside the body. The system produces its immune cells, chemical mes-sengers, and antibodies in the thymus, bone marrow, tonsils and adenoids, lymph nodes and vessels, spleen, skin and liver, mean-while allowing healing to occur as necessary.

During this acute inflammatory state, associated metabolic system effects can occur, such as lethargy, poor appetite, social withdrawal, and also a degree of insulin resistance. After contain-ing the problem, the immune system facilitates the remodelling and restructuring of damaged tissues, and then resolution occurs as the system returns to surveillance duties. All this can take several days. Usually, a memory is created so a repeat attack by the same intruder will provoke an immediate antibody response. As we age or become obese, unhealthy, or frail, our immune system deteriorates, making it easier for mutated cells or infection-causing germs to overwhelm the body's responses. However, under certain circumstances, there is prevention of the resolution phase, resulting in a state of chronic, low-grade, non-infective inflammation that tends to affect the whole body. These circumstances include social, psychological, environmental, and internal body processes.

Excessive fat tissue accumulation – that is, obesity – is also a promoter of systemic chronic inflammation. This state is associated with the development of metabolic syndrome and all the previously mentioned chronic diseases, as well as autoimmune diseases (thyroid and arthritis disorders).

CHRONIC STRESS

You may be familiar with the acute stress response. Faced with an imminent threat, like an attack by a large dog, or a house invader, there is an instant total-body response. Your body and mind are immediately on alert to 'fight or flee'. Hormones like adrenaline, noradrenaline, and cortisol influence the autonomic (automatic) nervous system, referred to as the sympathetic system. Your heart rate and blood pressure rise quickly, and fuel in your muscles is made available for rapid deployment. These acute stress effects are a feature of the sympathetic nervous system (its opposite, the calming system, is dominated by the parasympathetic system). These acute stress hormones counteract the effects of insulin, leaving plenty of glucose in the system for rapid energy production.

However, the realities of modern life have introduced a response called chronic stress, which occurs at different grades or levels. For example, a row with your partner will elicit a stress response, as will congestion in traffic or pressures at work. Living in fear at home, being anxious, being in deprivation, in poverty, being homeless or being threatened with homelessness, having poor food security, a chronically sick family member – any or all will cause a chronically activated stress pathology in the body. The various responses of the body include the production of numerous proteins, which demands high energy. As a result, energy is diverted from some of the body's other needs like house-keeping activities and restoring normality during rest and sleep, and the sympathetic system continues to dominate the parasym-pathetic system.

Another result is the release of molecules called cytokines, which trigger the chronic inflammatory state. When stress is chronic, the antagonistic effect on insulin is countered by increased production from the pancreas. This, in effect, is equiv-alent to insulin resistance. And so, the triad of insulin resistance (metabolic dysfunction), chronic inflammation, and chronic stress carry out a combined attack on health function.

I discuss recovery in the next chapter. Deep rest, contemplative practices, sporting or other enjoyable activities carried out in an environment of safety, with an experience of acceptance, belonging, and inclusion, may downgrade activation of the sympathetic system and restore calm.

PREVENTION PLAYBOOK
CHAPTER SUMMARY

Regarding the development of chronic diseases, it is difficult to decipher which comes first. However, it is clear that metabolic dysfunction, systemic chronic inflammation, and chronic stress impact each other and homeostasis, and are major contributors to all chronic disease outcomes.

Chapter 5

FOUR PILLARS THAT SUPPORT GOOD HEALTH

Caring for your body should be as natural as caring for a beautiful garden, or an expensive car, or a partner you adore.

I feel we are inclined to take our bodies for granted. It's exactly what I do with computers. You may be the same. Unless you are very familiar with computer technology, exactly how they work is of less interest than taking advantage of the fact that they work so well. While you are competent with the software and the keyboard, unless you are a computer engineer, those little circuits are of little interest. And when the computer doesn't work so well, you take it to an expert and are grateful when it is fixed. You may even fall asleep during the technician's explanation of what went wrong!

Similarly with our bodies, as long as we wake up in the morning and can get on with the day's activities, we are adequately satisfied. Even so, most of us will have occasional short-term health issues, like an infection or an injury, and will require assistance from a healthcare practitioner. The effects of aging will occur in everyone, but it is probable that we can slow down the process. Unfortunately, as I have inferred already, too many people develop chronic health issues that accelerate the aging process. Their overall health declines, and they become dependent on the healthcare system for consultations, tests, medications, hospitalisation, or surgery. When it becomes too difficult to cope from day to day, many people require home or residential care for years before they die.

Everyone should take an active interest in their health by becoming aware of what supports good healthy functioning of their cells and body. Fortunately, learning how to maintain good health is quite easy.

NEGOTIATING THE 'HEALTH' SPECTRUM

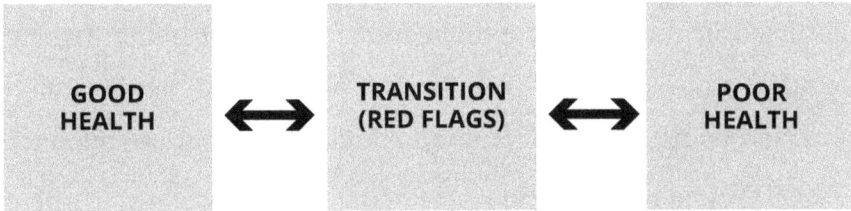

| GOOD HEALTH | ⟷ | TRANSITION (RED FLAGS) | ⟷ | POOR HEALTH |

When you take on personal responsibility for your health, becoming aware of what is required for your body and mind to function at their best will give you a clear appreciation of what drives human health. In contrast, ignoring the body's required supports, or adopting lifestyle behaviours that actively overwhelm its systems, is likely to lead to poor health. Increasingly, we are recognising these disease drivers.

> **The efforts required to support the health of your body are the same as those that are likely to give you long-term health and reduced risk of developing the commonest chronic diseases, which are responsible for so much dependence on the healthcare system and the unfortunate occurrence of premature death.**

At this point, it is important to acknowledge that not all poor health outcomes can be recognised or prevented, for example, genetic diseases, some cancers in children, some heart attacks, some strokes, and type 1 diabetes. It is sad when we hear about an apparently fit and 'healthy' person being diagnosed with a serious medical event or even premature death. My own story discussed in the final chapter demonstrates that being 'fit and healthy' is not a guarantee of perfect health, and regular metabolic screening from mid- to late-30s can highlight the need for proactivity.

On the positive side, I believe that if you invest the effort to achieve good health, you will reduce the risks of developing type 2 diabetes, heart diseases, and more. If you are 'lucky' to have good health, it is worthwhile understanding how to maintain it. If any of the Red Flag conditions (discussed in chapter seven) are noticed by you or diagnosed by your doctor, you can take steps to prevent deterioration and transition to poor health. If you have had a chronic disease already diagnosed, understanding what your body requires will help you heal.

Understand these two basic statements about your body:

1. On the assumption that the body will perform at its best if you support its functional requirements, you must be aware of what these are. I call these the *drivers of good health.*

2. Health can be negatively influenced by some choices you make, or external factors that are generally outside your control. You must be aware of these. I call these the *drivers of chronic disease.*

Your human body is an integrated whole that is dependent on its component parts – and it is mind-bogglingly complex. You could call it organised chaos! Not unlike the sight of thousands of people at a busy pedestrian crossing in Tokyo, or the murmuration of thousands of starlings creating their amazing sky dance, the activities inside the human body are ceaseless and fascinating at the same time.

The cells, tissues, glands, and organs are interconnected by a vast array of hormones, chemical messengers, neurotransmitters and modulators, immune cells, and growth factors that attach themselves to specific receptors on the surface of every cell. All these systems combine to generate your physical, emotional, and mental activities. Maintaining cellular and whole-body healthy function will optimise your health span. Pain experienced anywhere in your body creates a mental reaction, like sadness or frustration. Anxiety may be considered a mental state, yet it is often associated with physical responses like a racing heart and shortness of breath. It is impossible to isolate a body event from the mind, and vice versa.

THE FOUR SUPPORT PILLARS OF GOOD HEALTH

1. Nourishment
2. Movement
3. Recovery (sleep and deep rest/self-restoration)
4. Engagement (social and with nature), connectedness, and purpose

I could include sun exposure as well because of its important role in assisting the body produce vitamin D (with the aid of cholesterol), which in turn helps calcium absorption for stronger and healthier bones. However, I have decided to only give it a brief mention so we can focus on the other pillars, which require deeper explanation.

Let's take a closer look at the four pillars that sustain and maintain the body in the best possible health for the longest possible time. Can you plan to make these a daily part of your life?

1. Nourishment

Nourishment is the food (and water) necessary for life, growth, repair, and health. Exactly which food and drinks give the healthiest support to the body's functions is highly contentious.

However, recent lessons learnt from nutrition management of type 2 diabetes are slowly resolving the issue.

Food provides two essential ingredients for life: energy and nutrients.

Food Provides Energy – the Fuel of Life

We discussed some aspects of energy in chapter three. Here, I expand on that topic.

As mentioned, just like every other living organism, humans need a source of energy, continuously, every single moment, from before birth to our very last breath. Without that uninterrupted supply of energy, no human can exist.

All multicellular living organisms, plants, animals including humans, fish, birds, and insects exist directly or indirectly because of the sun. The sun may be one great big fireball in the sky, but it has a supreme impact on the existence of life on Earth. It is a powerful nuclear reactor emitting radiation energy to us earthly inhabitants. In its core, positively charged particles of hydrogen called protons bombard one another at great speed, emitting large quantities of energy.

Energy is not actually a physical, touchable thing. It is not made from something else. It is a capacity, or force, that exists in chemical bonds between elements like hydrogen, carbon, or phosphorous. Energy cannot be created or destroyed, but it can be transformed from one form to another. Solar energy radiates through space at the speed of light and comes to Earth as light, infrared energy – mostly felt as heat – and ultraviolet energy, which is the nasty stuff that gives us sunburn when skin is exposed too long to the sun. Not only does this solar energy impact all living organisms on Earth in one way or another, but it also influences our day and night, our winds and cyclones, and our ocean tides. It is little wonder that the sun was revered as a god in many societies.

Solar energy can be converted by plants to a usable form that allows them to grow, survive, and reproduce. Herbivores, like cattle, sheep, goats, and pigs (technically omnivores), can convert the energy from the plants they eat into usable forms to support their life cycles. Humans are omnivores and convert the energy contained in plants and animals into the human-usable form of energy called ATP.

Food Provides Essential Nutrients

Food must supply certain essential nutrients for healthy bodily function, that is, amino acids and lipids (fatty acids), vitamins, and minerals. Some food choices can lack one or more of these essential molecules and result in compromised health (for example scurvy from vitamin C deficiency or goitre from iodine deficiency). Some nutrition choices are known to predispose to dysfunction in processes, network functions, or structures (for example, ultra-processed foods).

Herein lies the crux of whether you exist in good health or upset the body's systems and processes and trend towards poor health. In effect, the major driver of health that you can control is what you consume as food or fluid. The dilemma is − what constitutes the best food?

It is a major social concern that the most nutritious foods may not be available to you because of economic or political circumstances, or you may unintentionally undervalue the significance of certain food choices.

Despite the arguments about the dietary preferences of our human ancestors, it is clear that throughout recorded history, *Homo sapiens* have been omnivores (consuming plant- and animal-sourced foods). For millennia, our ancestors ate the animals and fish they hunted, and fruit, nuts, and seeds when available. From about 10,000 years ago, vegetables, grains, and legumes were introduced. During this time, fruit oils (for example, olive oil) and dairy products also became available. From the 1600s, sugar became available and was loved by the wealthy. Later, sugar became more readily available, and mass consumption started.

From the late 1800s, the process of making seed oils commenced using cotton seeds, and this was ramped up during World War II using soybeans. Low-fat, high-carbohydrate, highly processed factory foods entered the market in the 1970s and have gained immense popularity since.

Over the last 100 years or so, there has been an evolutionary dissociation between our DNA, which is extremely slow to adapt, and changes in the food we consume. Our bodies' systems, and particularly our mitochondria, have not adapted to the presence of high levels of glucose, fructose, and seed oils, much of which have occurred since recommendations to reduce saturated fats in our diets in the 1960s and 1970s. While these changes were initially introduced in the US, they have been adopted in other parts of the world. In addition, the globalisation of major food corporations has contributed greatly to this problem. Present dietary advice and changes to our food production and choices have coincided with the increased prevalence of chronic diseases throughout the world.

Food is either sourced from nature (animal products, plant products) or is factory-made, producing highly refined processed or ultra-processed foods.

Who doesn't savour every last morsel of salt and vinegar potato chips? Who hasn't felt full after a lovely salad, only to find room for dessert? It is recognised that your food choices have varying satiety and addictive impacts. It is estimated that, in the US, people eat an average of around six times per day, including snacks.[1] Is this why their medical institutions estimate that almost 90 percent have evidence of metabolic dysfunction?[2] Many diabetes organisations suggest three main meals and two or three snacks meals per day. Surely, this is overloading an already strained metabolism. Considering that people adhering to low-carbohydrate or keto diets often find two meals per day to be adequately satiating, who is doing the best for their metabolic health?

There are intense debates regarding the potential make-up of what we might call optimal nutrition. As discussed earlier, some of the debates have presumed biases depending on the academic institution and the preference (or ideology) relating to the use or avoidance of animal foods. In some ways, this is sad because there is a broad agreement that the present food choices in many Western countries are clearly adding to poor health outcomes. For example, some researchers in the US refer in a derogatory manner to their prevailing diet as SAD (standard American diet)! Any change from present SAD nutrition choices offers an improvement in weight and other health markers. So, vegetarian, carnivore, low-carbohydrate, DASH (Dietary Approaches to Stop Hypertension), intermittent fasting, and the Mediterranean diets have all been shown to improve weight and health status, at least in the short term. The dietary battles rage because proponents of each of these dietary approaches are competing to be the number one option. In the background, of course, there are biases and commercial interests involved.

It is an unfortunate slight on food science research that one of the most respected analysts of medical scientific evidence (John Ioannidis from Stanford University) has reported that nutrition science is of very low quality and riddled with biases. In effect, the science of nutrition has been hijacked.

As we know, the recent literature demonstrates rapid successful remission of type 2 diabetes by adhering to low-carbohydrate, sugar-reduced nutrition. It seems reasonable from this to assume that your overall health will benefit from 'real food', just like in granny's youth, that is, food that has undergone little or no adulteration. Fresh, organic, seasonal fruit and vegetables and natural-environment meat, eggs, dairy, and fish. For some, this will mean eating as an omnivore, carnivore, or vegetarian. There is a rider, however. In the presence of metabolic dysfunction, it is wise to choose food that will reduce hyperinsulinaemia, which means adhering to a very-low-carbohydrate, ketogenic, or mostly carnivore diet.

2. Movement

A well-recognised 21st century change in human behaviour is the overall reduction in movement. It appears that each new generation is more sedentary than the previous one. Work practices these days involve sitting in front of a computer for hours on end, and evenings include too long in front of the television or engaging on social media. The exercise industries have found a niche. However, of the 6 million Australians who have a gym membership, only half attend once per week, and over 1 million go less than once per month.[3]

According to Peter Attia, internationally known doctor, podcaster, and author of *Outlive: The Science and Art of Longevity*, "Exercise has the greatest power to determine how you will live out the rest of your life."[4] A very big call! And he provides evidence that regular exercisers live as much as a decade longer than sedentary people.

Muscle mass decreases with aging, especially after age 65. With that decrease comes the potential for falls, immobilisation, and extreme loss of muscular ability and mobility. Consequently, a person's ability to perform the activities of daily life becomes compromised.

Unlike plants, humans have been made to move. Active muscles use up a lot of the energy that we get from food. Optimum exercise includes aerobic (for cardiorespiratory function) and resistance training (for muscle strength). Push-ups, leg squats, standing on one foot for 20 seconds can all be done today, and the benefits will come quite quickly. Depending on your level of fitness and mobility, walking, jogging, high-intensity interval training, resistance training, or a combination could become a regular part of your routine.

Exercise has a profound beneficial impact on mitochondria. It boosts their capacity to use food molecules for energy production, and it increases mitochondrial numbers. The exercise level called zone 2 (60 to 70 percent of maximum heart rate − able to carry out a conversation while jogging) may be the most effective at improving mitochondrial function.

To help you get started in the gym, a personal instructor or an exercise physiologist can get you assessed and organised. However, not all of us are interested in attending the gym or jogging. For those who aren't, as little as 2 minutes of walking multiple times each day gets muscles utilising glucose and improves metabolic status. Even a little regular activity negates the present-day tendency to be sedentary.

The benefits of exercise are beyond doubt and can be particularly enjoyable if done with friends or in class settings. As mentioned earlier, insulin is the important hormone to lower blood levels and deliver glucose into cells. The actual process is complex, as the insulin must attach to a cell's receptor, which in turn creates a channel for the glucose to enter. This process is faulty in people with pre-diabetes and type 2 diabetes. However, in exercisers, the requirement for insulin attaching to a cell receptor is not always required, and free admission of glucose into the cell occurs, giving the energy boost as required.

There are some authors who rate exercise as the most important factor for a long and healthy life. I agree on its importance, but I have already emphasised your body's need for good nutrition to give it the energy and essential macro and micronutrients it requires to exercise effectively. Obviously, the loss of mobility for whatever reason is a severe impediment to independent living.

And so...

For those who lead a sedentary life,
exercise becomes a must.

While the debate around nutrition rages on, the benefits of exercise couldn't be clearer:

1. Exercise can reduce the rate of loss of muscle related to aging.[5]
2. Exercise can slow or reverse the rate of cognitive decline.[6]
3. Exercise performed regularly each week is associated with a longer lifespan.[7]
4. Exercise has benefits for mitochondria, resulting in better energy; therefore, it improves management of heart disease and diabetes, as equally as or possibly greater than medications.[8]

Unlike the difficulties encountered in interpreting nutrition research, Professor Ioannidis, whom I mentioned earlier, has shown that there are numerous research trials that show that exercise is as powerful as various medications at reducing mortality from coronary heart disease, pre-diabetes, diabetes, and stroke.

Fitness, as measured by how much oxygen you can use per minute (VO2 max), improves cardiorespiratory fitness. But also important is resistance training – lifting weights or doing weight-bearing exercises like push-ups and squats, which increase and maintain the muscle strength required to climb and descend stairs safely and play ball games with children, and later grandchildren, as you age. Indeed, the joy gained from exercising and its unquestionable benefits drive good health, both mental and physical.

Please don't ignore the body's need for mobility and independence, the ability to get out into nature without relying on a carer, still throw or kick a ball or swing a tennis racquet even into your 90s. What an inspiration you would be for your friends and family!

3. Recovery (Sleep and Restoration)

Quality Sleep Is Essential

"Sleep is a non-negotiable biological necessity."
– Dr Matthew Walker

With that one quote from the sleep guru, Dr Matthew Walker, I realised that sleep had to be one of the important determinants of good health. So, why is sleep so important? How long should you sleep? What if you have a career in obstetrics like I did and have major interruptions to sleep on a regular basis? Is shift work detrimental to health?

Sleep certainly is a biological necessity. It influences quality of life, psychological wellbeing, and behaviour, cognitive function, physical health, and public safety. It is a state of active unconsciousness. Active for the obvious reason that your heart and breathing need to continue functioning. Yet they require less energy than when you are awake. Importantly, during sleep, recovery and healing occur for mental and physical functions. It is a time of reduced heart rate and blood pressure. But brain function is very active during sleep. Cellular housekeeping gets a chance to clear away the by-products of the day's cell activities. It is stated to be a time when events of the day and learning are moved from short- to long-term memory. Unfortunately, the transfer of new experiences or knowledge to long-term memory is interfered with when adequate sleep is not possible. This is important for those who are studying for exams. Just a few days of poor sleep can push metabolic function towards dysfunction.

There are so many life factors that interfere with getting to sleep and staying asleep for the recommended 7 to 8 hours – from a crying baby, a snoring partner, fear for safety, an exam or work deadline, coffee, alcohol, screens, light, noise. The ideal of a good night's sleep can be so difficult to achieve. Then there are the real problems of sleep apnoea (often related to obesity) and insomnia. Finally, there is the difficult problem of sleep quality. Do you wake up refreshed? I know many people resort to sedation, but unfortunately sleeping pills can interfere with aspects of good sleep, like the various stages and depth of sleep.

People who are sleep-deprived get the munchies and gain weight more easily, and there are hormonal reasons for this. In addition, even the loss of one night's sleep can trigger the release of the stress hormones cortisol and adrenaline. These hormones, in turn, promote insulin resistance. Poor sleep hygiene is associated with increased risk for heart disease and stroke.[9]

So, what does Dr Walker advise? Sleep hygiene! Your body has a natural sleep-wake cycle, so try to create a regular sleep schedule.

- Try not to eat within the few hours before going to bed.
- Keep alcohol and coffee to low levels or avoid.
- Beware of staying up too late binge watching the latest big streaming show.
- Try a warm bath (Dr Walker is English, and I expect that for us Australians, during our hot summers, we would be better off with a cool shower).
- Make the bedroom as dark as possible or use an eye mask.
- Reduce noise (a partner who snores may need to move or seek help from a sleep clinic).
- Turn off notifications on your mobile phone and computer. This is your very special and vital restorative time, and it must not be disturbed.[10]

There are helpful sleep fact sheets available at sleephealth-foundation.org.au.

Time for Self-Restoration

Do you sometimes feel overwhelmed with the demands and responsibilities of your daily life? Children, partner, transport, work, meals, housekeeping, bills to be paid, too little sleep. When can you get a break to slow down, to smell the roses, to restore yourself? How are you going to find the time? For good mental and physical health, I believe finding time for self-restoration complements the benefits gained from sleep.

The mind involves our emotions, thoughts, memories, our sense of self, our attitudes and motivations, our conscious and subconscious states, and probably a lot more. The mind cannot be seen or dissected like the brain or heart. I read somewhere that we know more about outer space than we do about the mind. It remains an incompletely understood but vital part of us. We are whole when our minds and our physical selves are functioning adequately. Our level of health is dependent on the relative health of the whole body.

The experience of stress in daily life is common and is associated with prolonged activation of the fight-or-flight state (chronic stress and an outpouring of cortisol and adrenaline), the exact opposite of feeling safe and being relaxed. Self-restoration is the antidote to the toxic effects of worry and stress, and the evidence for the benefits is strong. It is so very important to find the time to do something that makes you feel relaxed, to restore your enthusiasm and energy to face the next day, to become distracted for a while from the problems of today and the worries about the future that build up and drag you down.

In addition, there is a problem regarding social media use by children and adults. For all the accepted usefulness of the digital age, there are downsides. We are exposed to all the traumas of the world; children are exposed to adult content; addiction to gaming is a problem. All of these provoke low-level stress for many people. Presently, Australian academics report that there are concerns over a dramatic increase in hospitalisations of under 14-year-old boys and girls for self-harm.[11] Internationally, there are parliamentary plans to limit the availability of internet to children.

Self-restoration can be achieved through contemplative practices, for example, meditation or yoga, which are mind-body exercises that can assist inner wellbeing. When carried out in a calm, quiet, and safe area, contemplative exercises are a distraction that can decrease distressing emotions, depression symptoms, and perceived fear and stress. Blood pressure drops as your body's systems enter a phase called deep rest. Deep rest allows the mind and body to escape into a happy place. How mentally uplifting it is for the spirit to spend time in natural surroundings like a garden or forest, to observe the flow of water in a stream or the rolling waves of the ocean.

Deep rest is a counter to the chronically elevated stress hormones that are part and parcel of modern life. 'Deep rest' is a hypothesis from a group of American psychologists whose thesis is that deep rest is a physiological and psychological state that creates a biological environment that allows for cellular restoration and improved mitochondrial function – somewhat like sleep.

Essential Oil Use as Part of Self-Restoration

Traditional methods of healthcare were used when I was young. Toothache was treated with clove oil, and blocked nose and other symptoms of a 'cold' were treated with Vicks vapour ointment (menthol, eucalyptus, camphor) rubbed on the chest. Of course, many of the pharmaceutical drugs in use today are the concentrated active ingredients of plants used historically for different maladies. Morphine, heroin, codeine, digitalis, caffeine, nicotine, and medicinal cannabis are present-day drugs obtained from plant extracts.

It has been estimated that humans can differentiate a trillion different scents. While sound and colours come to us in waveform, there is no such dimension to understand how we detect scents. Today, we use diffusers soaked with essential oils derived from plants or fruits to create a clean and relaxing feeling in rooms. Essential oils are used in cosmetics, perfumes, and pharmaceuticals, and can be used in food, beverages, and cleaning products. The oils can be used by inhalation, by mouth, or by topical skin absorption.

The use of essential oils derived from aromatic plants has a 5,000-year history, showing increasing use around the world. The growth of the pharmaceutical industry has overshadowed traditional treatments of diseases, although there is still a considerable interest in the medical benefits of essential oils. There are benefits that can be gained from personal use of essential oils that do not carry the potential side effects of medications. Whether they work as a placebo or with a truly therapeutic effect, there are an increasing number of studies appearing in journals confirming their value when combined with self-restoration activities like meditation, massage, and aromatherapy. Indeed, the Australian Therapeutic Goods Administration (TGA) has given approval for the use of pure essential oils for many conditions, including palliative care, anxiety, and depression.

4. Engagement, Connectedness, and Purpose

A hugely important need for healthy mind care is to have engagement, social interaction with family and friends, to be an accepted member of society, to have daily purpose, to be able to express opinions, argue about politics, play some social team sport. Personal involvement with others through safe socialisation is a fundamental component of good health. This presupposes the non-existence of oppression and deprivation.

In addition, engaging with the wonders of nature provides relaxation and psychological calm. A lovely garden or forest area, a walk on the beach watching the rolling waves, and the flow of water in a stream provide a wonderful distraction that lowers stress and improves mood.

OTHER DISEASE PREVENTION AND SCREENING PROGRAMS

There are also government-recommended disease prevention strategies. The immunisation program includes the numerous childhood vaccinations, and there are various vaccination options for adults, including influenza, shingles, and pneumo-coccal vaccines. Mostly, these are for at-risk individuals or for those over the age of 65. Screening programs exist for breast and bowel cancer, and there are private options for prostate and ovarian cancer.

Tobacco-exposure-related diseases have reduced since extensive education, taxation, and the restriction of smoking areas were introduced. Smoking, and let's include vaping, is not conducive to good health in the short or long term.

Additionally, the campaign to reduce skin cancers through reducing skin exposure to excessive UV sunlight has had benefits and is something to consider in your health-management strategy.

PREVENTION PLAYBOOK
CHAPTER SUMMARY

———————

By using the drivers of good health, by giving your
body the essential support it needs from nourishment,
movement, recovery, and engagement socially and
with nature, you will maintain or return to better
health. You are the best person to take control
of the factors that promote your good health.

"Unthinking respect for authority is the greatest enemy of truth."

– Albert Einstein

Chapter 6

DRIVERS OF
CHRONIC DISEASES

**Most chronic diseases emerge from
prolonged exposure to one or more
of a range of factors, and so they
are multifactorial in origin.**

All of us will die. A death certificate must contain an opinion as to the probable cause of death. 'Old age', 'died from natural causes', or cardiac or respiratory failure do not qualify as causes of death. They are considered mechanisms rather than causes. Pneumonia is often the final illness that overcomes the elderly, although, for most, one or more chronic diseases will also be present.

Despite the dedication of our health practitioners and the efforts of health policymakers, despite the regular reports of breakthroughs in one or another disease, despite being told we have the best healthcare system in the world, you know as well as I do that something isn't right.

National statistics here and elsewhere reveal a sorry tale. All chronic illnesses are becoming more frequent and are occurring even in younger age groups. Approximately 1 in 4 Australians have two or more chronic diseases that lower their quality of life for many years before they die.[1] Medications are prescribed for huge swathes of the population, so much so that there is concern about polypharmacy (the simultaneous use of five or more different medications). Confusion, mistakes, and drug interactions mean that long-term use of medications is a major contributor to hospital admissions and even death, especially in the elderly. Further, mental health disorders have become more frequent, with them being diagnosed in 39 percent of 16- to 24-year-old Australians overall, and as high as 46 percent among females.[2] It is of little wonder that the healthcare system is under stress.

Medical help is often not involved until an individual becomes concerned about some persisting symptoms. By the time an individual's health has deteriorated and the doctor diagnoses a chronic disease, there may already be some level of damage to one or more organs or tissues throughout the body. Early warning signs may have been missed (see chapter seven on health Red Flags). This applies particularly to heart diseases, type 2 diabetes, and dementia. Individuals and healthcare practitioners often do not recognise the underlying metabolic dysfunction that drives these conditions. Furthermore, there is increasing complexity when a second or third disease is diagnosed. This, coupled with ageing, frailty, and numerous medications – some with side effects – can leave individuals and their carers feeling frustrated and hopeless.

In addition, many routine blood results are said to be within the normal range; thus, reassurance is given, and no real action is taken. Upper-normal levels are not optimum! For example, upper-normal levels of liver enzymes probably indicate a degree of fatty liver change, which is an indicator of metabolic dysfunction, and preventative steps can improve the problem quite quickly. I discuss testing in chapter 13.

Many individuals will attend acupuncture and natural medicine practitioners to complement their conventional medical care. Complementary medicine (CM) holds a significant place alongside conventional medicine in caring for the medical needs of Australians. In Australia, more than one third of people have consulted with at least one CM practitioner, and over half have used a CM product or practice. These figures are about equivalent to estimated visits to doctors. Massage therapists, chiropractors, and yoga teachers were the most frequented (possibly because back pain affects so many people). Acupuncturists, naturopaths, osteopaths, and practitioners of traditional Chinese medicine were visited less frequently.[3]

The use of complementary medicine has been consistent over several surveys, suggesting that users are satisfied with the results. There is increasing evidence of the benefits of using acupuncture to address migraine, low back pain, and anxiety disorders, and using herbal medicines to address hormone conditions and delayed fertility.

* * *

When dealing with health and disease, everyone likes to break problems down into subsections, from which they can more easily categorise and understand what the major contributors to poor health are. Disease occurrence is influenced by an array of genetic and personal risk behaviours, as well as environmental, political, social, economic, and commercial factors.

From the mid-1900s to now, there has been a gradual increase in longevity. While there are more older Australians, the incidence of chronic diseases appears to be increasing at a greater rate, causing a tsunami of individuals dependent on the medical system.

Attempts at understanding the causes of these chronic diseases have involved epidemiologists, the medical science professions, and governmental public health policymakers.

DISEASE – A TRIP THROUGH HISTORY

From the distant past to now, humans have grappled with the

causes of poor health and premature death. Certainly, infections, especially in childhood, injuries from battle, accidents, and starvation all took an enormous toll. Otherwise, causes of disease were thought to be due to being possessed by demons or the devil, punishment by the gods for misdeeds, bad air in swampy areas, or imbalance in the 'four humours' of Hippocrates (black bile, yellow bile, phlegm, blood).

The invention of the microscope in the 1670s allowed the observation of microorganisms. By the late 1800s, Louis Pasteur and Robert Koch had recognised bacteria and evolved the 'germ theory', where they showed that one type of germ was the cause of a specific disease. Examples include leprosy, syphilis, cholera, typhoid, tuberculosis, and puerperal fever.

During the same era, certain disorders, such as scurvy, were found to be due to a deficiency of an item identified in food – vitamins (in the case of scurvy, there was a vitamin C deficiency). Following on from the vitamin knowledge, the search for the cause of certain diseases, like heart disease, fostered a new sub-branch of research called epidemiology, which sought to find associations between various lifestyle factors and diseases. Lung cancer was found to be associated with cigarette smoking. However, nutritional epidemiology has become a minefield of borderline findings that have exaggerated the benefit or danger of some foods. Eggs are a great example. Eggs are good for you; eggs are bad for you, which study do you believe?

Meanwhile, as our understanding grew in the fields of anatomy (structure, organs, and so on), physiology (the roles played by the various organs), and biochemistry (all those chemical reactions, enzymes, hormones, red and white blood cells, and so on), the body became understood in the context of a machine with parts that functioned well in good health. When they malfunctioned, attention could then be given to correcting the organ at fault.

Conventional medicine has evolved from general practitioners to specialists and even super-specialisation. Specialist doctors' daily work is dependent on which body system may be malfunctioning, the system they have spent years training in, whether it be as a surgeon (orthopaedic; cardiac; brain; generalist; ear, nose and throat; ophthalmologist; urologist; gynaecologist; endocrinologist; cardiologist; pulmonary physician; anaesthetist; intensivist; oncologist; and so on). Of course, there are also specialists in disorders of the brain and mental illness, neurologists, neurosurgeons, and psychiatrists.

This silo approach to poor health and disease has many benefits. However, we forget that humans are more than the organ in trouble. The whole body has highly integrated systems where every part communicates with the rest. Our minds, our emotions, our arthritis or appendicitis affect the whole body. As a result, integrative and holistic medical practitioners have become more common.

IT'S TIME TO TALK ABOUT OBESITY...

Every human needs to have some fat in their diet and fat tissue in their body. Fat is an active tissue, constantly turning over its stores. It has important roles in the body, for example, energy storage and release, cushioning around organs, insulation from both cold and heat, and more. It is obvious when comparing males and females that sex hormones determine where fat is stored.

When fat is present in excess, it is related to many health issues. This is particularly true if the fat accumulates around the abdominal organs (referred to as central or visceral fat), in the liver (fatty liver), and in the pancreas. If obesity is diagnosed, it is likely that other organs, like the heart and kidneys, will have extra fat around them, which may impair their function. Furthermore, various government strategic plans for the health of Australians recognise that prevention and management of obesity are worthwhile goals. Weight loss of about 5 percent is associated with improvement in chronic disease markers.[4]

Body mass index (BMI) is the measurement used to differentiate between weight categories. The BMI formula is your weight divided by your height squared (weight / height^2).[5]

Body Mass Index Ranges

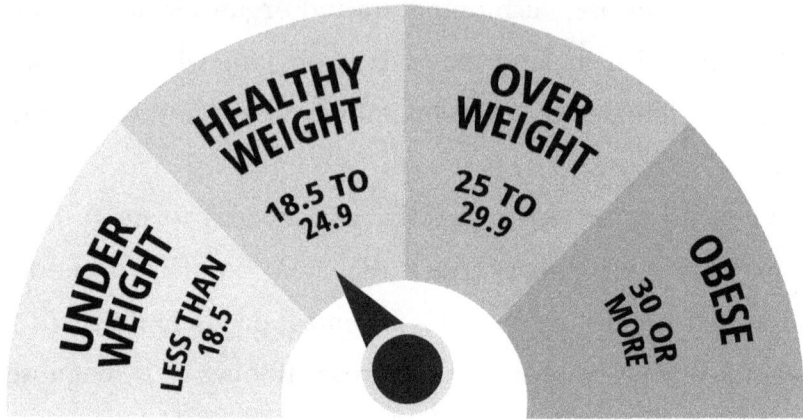

Other indexes are also used to categorise obesity, such as waist circumference, waist-to-height ratio, and waist-to-hip ratio.

Current average adult weight is about 15 kg heavier compared to the 1960s. In Australia, obesity rates have been steadily trending upwards for decades.[6]

Is Obesity a Disease?

Yes, according to the World Health Organization, the American Medical Association, the Centers for Disease Control, and various Australian Government reports, obesity is a disease. In 2018, obesity was added to the Australian list of medical conditions eligible for the Chronic Disease Management Scheme, and Medicare item numbers have been included to provide patients with financial support.[7] National statistics recognise that 32 percent of Australians have a BMI greater than 30 (obese), and another 34 percent are considered overweight, meaning 66 percent of adults are outside of the healthy normal range. In addition, 25 percent of children are overweight or, frankly, obese.[8] The figures are higher in rural Australia.

Obesity impacts all levels of society, from poverty to affluence. The conditions of overweight and obesity are increasing rapidly. A minority of individuals who are obese have no blood markers or other markers of metabolic dysfunction – at least for a while. They are described as having metabolically healthy obesity (MHO). However, with the passage of time, this state is very likely to progress to chronic poor health.

Why Is There Concern About Obesity?

About 30 different diseases are related to being overweight or obese. There are the well-recognised chronic diseases, such as type 2 diabetes, hypertension, heart disease, stroke, and chronic kidney disease. Also, there are 13 different cancers significantly related to the presence of obesity. Additionally, problems of daily living include sleep apnoea, reflux (gastroesophageal reflux), mobility issues related to osteoarthritis, and the embarrassment of urinary incontinence. Further, later life cognitive dysfunction due to dementia is increased due to obesity-related metabolic dysfunction.

What Causes a Person to Become Overweight?

That is a million-dollar question...

Remember, food must supply all the macro and micronutrients we need to fuel the energy requirements of every cell and support bodily processes, like heartbeat, breathing, brain processes, and to provide the building blocks for growth, maintenance, repair, and reproduction throughout our lives. So, where does it all go wrong? There are two main theories that shed some light on the probable causes of overweight and obesity: the energy balance model (EBM) and the carbohydrate-insulin model (CIM).

Energy Balance Model (EBM) of Obesity

The EBM focuses on how much energy we consume versus how much energy we expend.

In the normal physiological state of a lean person, there is a dynamic balance (homeostasis) between the energy (measured in calories) we consume from food, the energy we make, use, and store (as glycogen and fat), and the amount of nutrients required to maintain every cell and tissue activity, such as growth and repair, whether sedentary or exercising.

> **It is extraordinary to realise that a daily increase in excess fat storage of just 1 gram per day from age 20 (less than the energy in one teaspoon of sugar) can tip a person into the obese category by age 35.**

Really? Do we have to be that careful to not consume an excess of just one teaspoon of sugar or its equivalent per day? For the most part, energy balance is dependent on three important items: the quality of the food we eat, the quantity of food, and the efficiency of the metabolic processes in our bodies.

Food Quality

The NOVA food classification system distinguishes foods depending on the amount of processing carried out before they can be consumed. In essence, there are recognisable real foods, which are foods as nature intended, that are low-energy and nutrient-dense (meat, fish, dairy, nuts, fresh vegetables and fruit, and whole grains). Alternatively, there are refined, highly processed, high-energy, nutrient-poor foods, with their excess sugar, seed oil fats, salt, and a host of other chemicals. Because highly refined and processed foods and drinks are hyperpalatable, cheap, convenient, and readily available, overconsumption is common. Think sugar drinks, ice cream, cakes, biscuits, breakfast cereals, fast foods, and many foods that, to paraphrase professor and author Benjamin Bikman, are boxed, bagged, and carry a barcode.

Food Quantity

Overconsumption and a sedentary lifestyle will eventually result in weight gain and metabolic dysfunction. Overconsumption can be partly compensated for with physical activity. This knowledge led to the emphasis on food's caloric values and the calorie counting craze, where calorie intake should be countered by calorie expenditure. People were advised to eat less and move more in an effort to maintain the energy balance mentioned previously. Thus, when a person becomes overweight or obese, the fault is placed squarely on the individual's shoulders rather than on the food industries. A friend likened this attitude of blaming the consumer for overconsumption to the American gun lobby who state that it is not the gun that kills — it's the person pulling the trigger!

Carbohydrate Insulin Model (CIM) of Obesity

The CIM focuses on what our bodies do with what we eat.

It is the overriding duty of insulin to manage the amount of glucose (carbohydrates) that enters the bloodstream after a meal. When dietary experts suggested that the human diet should be 50 to 60 percent carbohydrates spread over 3 to 6 meals per day, insulin production by the pancreas became greater than ever in human history, rarely going back to minimal blood levels during the day. Eventually, cells become resistant to insulin's action to reduce blood glucose levels, causing a compensatory increased production of insulin by the pancreas.

Insulin has other significant functions beyond managing blood glucose levels in the body. It is also a growth hormone; it creates preferential conversion of glucose to the lipid triglyceride, and it prevents the release of fat for use as fuel. As a result, some tissues are left in an energy deficit, which activates the body's survival mechanisms, promoting feelings of hunger and leading to further food consumption. Overconsumption is the outcome.

Obesity Management Options

People with obesity who lose 5 percent or more body weight often – but not always – show improvement in mental and physical health outcomes, including blood markers. And so, there is a big interest and investment in the science and practice of measures to control excessive weight.

Bariatric surgery, which reduces the capacity of the stomach so overconsumption becomes impossible, has been enormously important for two reasons. Firstly, most people benefit from considerable and prolonged weight loss. Secondly, it became evident that type 2 diabetes and hypertension associated with obesity can be improved rapidly after surgery, and diabetes and blood pressure medications can be reduced or even ceased.

Very-low-calorie diets (about 800 kcal per day instead of the average 2500 to 3000 kcal per day) also work for weight loss and improving type 2 diabetes but have considerable problems related to hunger, motivation, and compliance, with many abandoning the diet and suffering considerable weight gain subsequently.

Recently available diabetes drugs for treating type 2 diabetes (Ozempic, Wegovy, Mounjaro) that have the bonus of weight loss influence the body's metabolism, reducing the absorption of food, enhancing hormones that promote insulin production, or prompting satiety within the gut, liver, and brain. They have been recorded with weight loss of 15 to 20 percent from starting weight.[9] However, they are expensive, require injections, and sometimes have intolerable or serious side effect potentials. Yet when the potential benefits outweigh the nuisance of minor side effects and the small potential for serious side effects, they can be an important resource.

Low-carbohydrate nutrition... Since the breakthrough in understanding metabolic dysfunction and its successful correction when limiting sugars (drinks and foods with added sugar), starches (potatoes, rice), and refined grains (flour), many people living with type 2 diabetes have been able to reduce or cease medications for diabetes and hypertension and successfully lose considerable weight. Rather than considering low-carbohydrate, keto, time-restricted eating, or fasting as 'diets', proponents believe they should be thought of more as ways of eating than as diets. They believe that these 'ways of eating' are successful in the long term because they are associated with satiety, and they are sustainable.

Of course, exercise also helps. But, as is often stated, "You can't outrun a bad diet." More exercise is often accompanied by more food consumption. For some, however, commencing an exercise program marks the beginning of a focus on overall health, which includes better eating habits and avoidance of other lifestyle risks.

While these various forms of obesity management are associated with significant weight loss, returning to consumption of high-energy sugars and starches must be avoided; otherwise, rapid weight regain will occur.

All approaches to weight loss rely on continued effort. For those who are concerned about being overweight, it may be better to develop a health focus (positive goal of eating better, exercising, aiding recovery through better sleep and deep rest, and engaging in socialisation), rather than a weight loss focus (which can become restrictive, create cravings and upset, and eventually lead to a negative outcome).

Can Obesity Be Prevented?

Scientists researching overweight and obesity and their causes will continue their debates into the future. It appears that most diets will give at least short-term benefits, although individuals' persistence becomes a problem, and weight regain is common. As mentioned, treatment options for established obesity are available.

Would prevention be better than attempting treatment later after the problem and its related health outcomes have become an issue? The answer, of course, is yes.

Obesity is mostly a metabolism problem related to food quality, quantity, and the presence of insulin resistance and hyperinsulinaemia. Additionally, some foods trigger reward centres in the brain, creating food addiction issues.

In Australia, there is no recommendation regarding sugar intake for children. The American Heart Association suggests that children should consume less than 25 grams, or six teaspoons, of added sugar per day, and the World Health Organization recommends that no more than 10 percent of overall calories come from added sugar.[10]

I believe there should be no added sugar in children's diets — but I admit I don't have to have those discussions with children who are fed double or triple that amount at every birthday party they go to!

The Australian Government, through its Department of Health and Aged Care, recognises that the government must increase its involvement in prevention as well as management of obesity. There are many possible strategies available, including improving citizens' nutrition literacy and potentially influencing food manufacturers to better label their products. The government also recognises that there are problems with the Health Star Rating system, which is presently voluntary for food producers and is not a reliable indicator of the health benefits or harms.

So, what can you do to support normal functioning of your body and thereby reduce your risk of developing one of the chronic diseases? Chapter 13 discusses how to establish your own personal goals and wishes regarding your health, tests that you can do to reveal your present state of health, and some straightforward and clear tips to aid your success.

GENETIC DRIVERS OF POOR HEALTH

It seems to be hardwired in humans to try and understand the workings of nature. Such enquiry led to the present theories about how the body functions normally and what causes the various maladies. This involved many brilliant people from many different eras and disciplines. However, it sometimes seems like the more you know, the more you don't know. Nevertheless, the quest goes on to continually bring our knowledge to a level that may benefit mankind. Unfortunately, some avenues of research may go down many unhelpful rabbit holes and be unproductive, and some knowledge may have commercial rather than honest scientific aims.

The importance placed on genetics probably started with the appreciation of inheritance as recognised by Mendel in the mid-1800s, even though there was no understanding of genes at that time. He noted that certain traits were inherited from our ancestors, for example, eye colour and height. Subsequent advancements in science have revealed that the smallest basic unit of the human body is the cell – and there are trillions of them. Inside the cell is a dominant feature called the nucleus. It is made up of DNA, the molecule of genetic inheritance.

You may have heard that in 1953 the structure of DNA was described as a three-dimensional double helix that contained the coding for creating a human, distinct from any other living organism.

We discovered that humans have 23 sets of chromosomes, which are recognisable under a powerful microscope just before a cell divides. Each chromosome has two arms, one from the mother and the second from the father. Numerous health problems have been identified that are a direct result of numerical or structural problems with one chromosome or another. For example, there can be too many chromosomes, like in Down syndrome where there are three arms of chromosome number 21, referred to as trisomy 21. Others include trisomy 18 and trisomy 13. Females have two X sex chromosomes, while males have one X and one Y sex chromosome. Various patterns have been identified, for example, XXY and XXX. Also, there can be an absence on one chromosome arm; for example, in Turner's syndrome, the chromosome complement is 45X.

Genes are the basic unit of heredity, and each chromosome contains thousands of these structures. The total complement of genes is called the genome, and a massive global effort was undertaken to map it. It is reasonable to assume that if the genes and chromosomes are perfectly normal in every way, then that lucky individual human will also be perfect. However, this is not the case, and most of us will have some variation in our gene pool even though we may appear normal and be in good health.

When over 90 percent of the Human Genome Project was completed in 2003 (finally completed in 2022), it was thought that we would be able to identify the genetic sequence variations that would give rise to all chronic diseases, including cancer. Certainly, the cause of some diseases can be traced to a single gene defect in an individual. Examples include cystic fibrosis, spinal muscular atrophy, and fragile X syndrome. There are some families that carry a very high risk of developing breast or ovarian cancer and carry a single gene defect called BRCA1 or BRCA2. There are about 2,000 known single gene (monogenic) variants that can cause disease. Screening for the presence of up to 500 of these variations is presently available to parents planning a pregnancy. Most perfectly healthy individuals will have a few single gene variations and will never suffer from the genetic change. They are carriers of the defect. If the identical variations are also found in the partner, there will be a 25 percent chance of passing the affected gene variation on to their child, who will develop the associated disorder.[11] Sometimes the clinical signs related to the disorder may be obvious to specialists soon after birth, yet for many the features of the single gene defect will not become apparent for years.

When scientists were getting closer to understanding the DNA and genetic causes of poor health, political enthusiasm reached the point of overreaction, and the US declared a 'war on cancer', with the hope of beating the disease within 5 years. Well, we know that, 50 years later, cancer remains a serious cause of poor health and premature death despite a massive investment in research and numerous wonderful developments in science, accompanied by advances in computing technology. Over 1,000 genes have been linked to cancer and are classified as cancer-associated genes.

Likewise, it was thought that obesity and all the chronic diseases, like diabetes, coronary vascular diseases, and rheumatoid arthritis, and various mental health disorders, like major depression, autism, ADHD, bipolar disorder, and Alzheimer's disease, were dependent on our genes, and to a certain extent that is true. However, there are tens of genetic variants that are associated with each of the chronic disorders. So again, drivers of disease are usually multifactorial, combining some genetic predisposition and environmental, behavioural, and lifestyle factors. A genetic predisposition can influence the onset, severity, and prognosis of the chronic conditions.

However, as we shall see, after enormous research time, effort, and expenditure, it is now clear that our genetics contribute only about 10 to 20 percent to cancers and other chronic diseases. The remainder is due to other factors like the environment and human behaviour.

The scientific developments in genetics have not been in vain. The potential to use genetic markers to recognise serious illnesses before they manifest clinically, and the use of genetic therapies, have tremendous future potential.

While not strictly related to genetics, I am intrigued by pregnancy and the potential for chronic non-communicable diseases to be related to events during this amazing 9-month period, in particular how the pregnant woman's personal safety, nutrition, medications, drugs, alcohol use, and smoking (add vaping also) can impact the developing baby. The vulnerability of a baby during pregnancy has been demonstrated repeatedly for decades. There were terrible outcomes for babies whose mothers were prescribed or took medications during pregnancy, for example, thalidomide (for pregnancy sickness), diethylstilboestrol (to prevent miscarriage), more recently valproate (anti-epilepsy medication), and a progestin hormone medication to 'diagnose pregnancy'. In addition, large intakes of alcohol during pregnancy can have a drastic effect on the developing baby (fetal alcohol syndrome).

mRNA vaccines were mandated for pregnant women during the pandemic, and I am very concerned about their potential impact on babies.. When one realises the growth rate of cells in a baby (200,000 new brain cells every minute at 20 weeks gestation) and their vulnerability to undergo some level of mutation, I believe no new or novel medications should be given to pregnant women.

It will be of no great surprise that it has been of great interest to me in my career as an obstetrician to follow the development of a hypothesis called the 'fetal origins of adult disease', originally coined by Professor David Barker, an English epidemiologist. Knowing that most infant mortality in the 1930s occurred within 1 week of birth and these deaths were usually associated with over or undernutrition, he assumed that there were adverse events influencing the growth and development of the baby during pregnancy. Even though Barker recognised that other potential causes like nutritional stores of iron and other micronutrients, stress, and hypoxia could be associated with low birth weight, undernutrition was the likely problem. His team then looked at death rates from heart disease in several districts in England and noted the correlation between low birth weight and premature death later in life from heart disease and stroke.

This 'fetal origins' hypothesis (while not genetic as such), which proposes that events during pregnancy influence later life chronic diseases, was borne out in several countries and has morphed into a whole field of medicine called the 'developmental origins of health and disease'. We now believe that the period of pregnancy may be the most influential and consequential 9 months in a human life.

The potential for events during pregnancy to exert influence on later life health has been borne out by other events. For example, after the 1918 flu pandemic, it was found that babies whose mothers had the flu during pregnancy were much more likely to develop disabling conditions, such as severe kidney disorders and schizophrenia.[12]

When the German blockade of Holland for 3 months from November 1944 caused pregnant women to eat only one third of their normal daily food, their babies developed subsequent problems. Babies who were still in the first trimester during the blockade were more likely to develop hypertension, obesity, and type 2 diabetes.[13] Those who were in the third trimester during the famine were born small and remained smaller than average for the remainder of their lives.[14]

Methods for altering genes are being actively researched. It is possible to use genetic methods to identify early disease states, help identify the most useful medication to treat an individual's disease, and modify genes to treat or cure disease. There are genetic engineering techniques to replace a disease-causing gene with a healthy copy, or to turn off a problem gene. This is all in the realm of personalised medicine.

I remain excited about future developments in genetic technology. However, my mantra is as previously stated – be aware of what promotes good health, and be aware of the drivers of poor health you can control. This gives you the knowledge of how you can prevent chronic diseases, and indeed help your body return to a healthier state if you have been unfortunate enough to develop a chronic medical condition.

LIFESTYLE DRIVERS OF POOR HEALTH

Lifestyle drivers of poor health are the day-to-day lifestyle choices people make that are known to be associated with the common chronic diseases like heart disease, diabetes, dementia, and cancer. And so, if you recognise that some of your lifestyle choices are known to contribute to poor health outcomes, you may take action to avoid or curtail these.

It is certain that poor health will eventually develop if the requirements of the body that drive good health are not met. To recap, your body needs good food choices, adequate exercise and sleep, caring for your mental health through contemplative practices, engagement with others and with nature, including some sun exposure to facilitate vitamin D production, and adhering to recommended preventative advice like cancer screening and immunisations.

These are general statements, easy to make, but as they say, the devil is in the detail! What are healthy food choices? How much and what type of exercise do you need? How many hours of sleep and how much sunshine do you need?

Smoking, Vaping, Illegal Recreational Drugs

I have a strong bias against smoking and vaping. The health risks are well-recorded.

Recreational drugs are illegal. No further discussion. There is strong evidence that mood altering drugs are associated with health and societal issues.

Alcohol

There is little doubt that excessive consumption of alcohol is detrimental to long-term health. But what is excessive?

Everyone knows that abuse of alcohol has multiple consequences for the individual, family, and wider social circles. However, should we consider the 'safe' consumption of alcohol a risk behaviour, and therefore recommend its avoidance? Should the WHO and other authorities apply their fear of alcohol to other risk behaviours like driving a car (should we only drive once per day and less than four times per week?), playing golf (golf cart accidents, errant golf balls, flying clubs), partaking in sport, (66,500 hospitalisations for sports injuries per year in Australia), jogging on the road, snow skiing holidays?[15] Are we being overprotected?

Alcohol is not a requirement of a healthy functioning body. There is no essential dietary requirement for alcohol (actually, the same is true for carbohydrates and sugar). But can it be part of self-restoration, time for you, your partner, and friends to relax together, part of the social interactions that are requirements for every human? These points are rarely considered by anti-alcohol proponents.

Let's now look at the negatives.

Just like many hormones and chemicals in the human body, and every single pharmaceutical medication that is prescribed, there is a dose-related effect. Alcohol is given priority status by the liver, as it is viewed as a toxin. Alcohol freely crosses into the brain and exerts effects from the ethanol, as well as histamines and nitrates (in wine), but also toxic by-products called acetaldehyde and acetate, which can be used as energy. Everyone knows that alcohol will cause headaches, sleep changes, mood alterations and behaviour changes, all the worse when taken in excess, including binge drinking. An individual's personal wellbeing is impacted for a considerable length of time after consuming an excess of alcohol. Additionally, drunken behaviour is responsible for social disharmony, domestic and other violence, and motor vehicle and work-related accidents.

Long-term excess – whatever that is – has been associated with weight gain, numerous cancers including breast cancer, heart disease including palpitations and arrhythmias, and liver disorders including fatty liver disease, cirrhosis, and cancer. Use in pregnancy at moderate to high levels is associated with fetal alcohol syndrome, a problem first described late last century, and a serious problem in Central Australia.

Alcohol may be combined with sweet additives and is often accompanied by eating nuts and carbs. Because of a relative short-term change in cells' insulin resistance, alcohol contributes to weight gain. It is also suggested that alcohol may cause gut permeability, allowing toxins and bacteria to get into the bloodstream.

The International Agency for Research on Cancer (IARC) has classified alcohol as a 'Grade 1' carcinogen, that is, the same bracket as asbestos and nicotine. In a hard-hitting 2022 press release, the WHO said there is no known safe level of alcohol consumption. In addition, risks start with the first drop.[16] In 2025, the US, Irish, and Australian governments proposed a need for producers to label their alcohol-containing products with warnings stating that alcohol can cause cancer.

The research that supports the statements by IARC and WHO are from epidemiological studies, where risks of cancer rise depending on the pure alcohol volume consumed per day. At worst, the relative risk of cancer is increased twofold from consumption of 100 g per day (equivalent to about 7 x 375 ml bottles of full-strength beer or one and a half 750 ml bottles of wine).[17] In comparison, the studies that condemned smoking cigarettes (nicotine) because of the relationship with lung cancer showed a 15 to 30 times increase in the relative risk of cancer development.[18] Epidemiologic studies are useful but cannot confirm causation, especially with low relative risk numbers. In addition, epidemiological studies are rarely able to differentiate one potential variable in a person's life from another as the causal factor. This is called confounding – a very common problem when 24-hour questionnaires are the basis of the data.

On the positive side, low to moderate consumption has been associated with lower risks of type 2 diabetes. However, the evidence suffers from the same confounding factors, that is, epidemiological studies (read more about alcohol in chapter 13).

Inactivity

I briefly discussed the benefits of exercise earlier in this chapter. Simply put, a sedentary lifestyle, whether self-imposed, work-related, or because of some chronic illness, is associated with shorter lifespan.

OTHER INFLUENCES ON HEALTH

Without health awareness, we become easy targets for those who wish to capitalise on our naivety.

Your health is also dependent on many major factors that are outside your control and are possibly more powerful than your own personal efforts to promote your health and avoid diseases. They are referred to as socio-economic, political, and environmental drivers of disease. These are determined to a major degree by governments and the business world.

The Australian government, through its health department and other funded organisations (for example, the NHMRC [National Health and Medical Research Council]), controls 'best-evidence' health guidelines (for example, Australian dietary guidelines), issues preventative strategies, and is responsible for the social, economic, and educational standards of the population.

Large business organisations in the food and pharmaceutical industries have commercial influences that can impact the overall health status of the country. Their involvement has advantages and disadvantages.

Of course, health practitioners, the caring professionals like nurses, doctors, dieticians, and others, are the coalface when we are concerned about our various maladies, and mostly we trust their recommendations. However, politics during the COVID pandemic influenced the top medical board (called AHPRA) to warn health practitioners to be aware that any advice given to patients against the COVID vaccines could result in disciplinary measures.[19] So, who controls medical knowledge? There are many influencers, as we shall see.

In truth, I have no personal experience in the sociopolitical manoeuvrings of health. However, I have read extensively over the years from government health strategies, dietary guidelines, and numerous revelations regarding the influence of big business over universities, governments, institutions, advocacy groups, and media. Background agendas and biases may conceal motives in guidelines and even journal articles. A working knowledge of critical analysis is essential to help one sift through the confusion of how best to attain good health and avoid poor health. It is important to be able to separate clever marketing claims from reality. When you are given advice by your healthcare practitioner, there is a lot to be gained by asking, "Why are you recommending this? How does it work? What are the benefits and risks? Is there an alternative? Please explain it so I can understand it better."

GOVERNMENT RESPONSIBILITY AND THE STATE OF DISEASE IN AUSTRALIA AND ABROAD

If you live in Australia, you live in a First World country. There is peace, no famine, no political oppression; we have clean running water; sanitation facilities are good; we are told we have a world-class medical system, and we have free access to healthcare through Medicare. Australians spend $252 billion per annum or nearly $10,000 per person on healthcare each year.[20] In theory, you should expect that we have a very healthy population. There has been a tendency to place the blame for obesity and the development of other poor health conditions on individuals' lifestyle choices and a lack of discipline – that is, they are self-inflicted. You can hear the authorities say, "Don't smoke or abuse alcohol, and eat plenty of fresh fruit, vegetables, grains, and legumes," but clearly it's not enough.

Somehow, it's not looking good for Australia! Our social system is failing and as sure as night follows day, so too will the health of our citizens. We have a well-recognised cost-of-living crisis, a housing crisis; our hospitals have ambulances ramping in line; there are long waiting lists for surgery; doctors and nurses are overworked; our aged-care industry is in turmoil, and we have thousands of families living in tents in parks and under bridges in our cities. The welfare organisations have not seen this level of concern before. Half the adult population has one or more mental or physical chronic illnesses, and many of them require multiple medications every day. These social and economic problems create chronic stress, health inequality, and for some the mental anguish of hopelessness.

As long ago as 1998, the World Health Organization director general affirmed that non-communicable chronic diseases were the major causes of poor health and death globally – more impactful than infections and wars. While there was an emphasis on the global community, he identified that all countries should take preventative action, as in any population most people have a moderate level of risk factors, and some have a high level. The WHO's 2023 report states that up to 41 million deaths occur annually from chronic diseases, with nearly half of these deaths occurring before age 70.[21]

Australia recognises that there are health disparities in the country. In addition, chronic diseases are common in all parts of the country; therefore, all citizens, whether in compromised or affluent areas, deserve the government's urgent attention to the worsening chronic disease crisis.

Societal and economic drivers of poor health are not only a concern in poverty-stricken countries in Africa. There are very real discrepancies in health outcomes in the UK, USA, and Australia. While average life expectancy in the UK is over 80 years, there is roughly a 9-year difference between individuals in well-off and less-well-off communities.[22] Life expectancy in the US is only 77 years, and 88 percent of the adult population have poor metabolic health.[23] In Central Australia, there is a diabetes crisis affecting 17 percent of Indigenous people.[24] Aboriginal women have one of the highest incidences of gestational diabetes in the world.[25] In that part of the country, the health system is being overwhelmed, and kidney dialysis clinics are at absolute capacity. Further, fetal alcohol syndrome and type 2 diabetes have been seen in children.

The mental health impacts from unaffordable housing and high food and energy prices are affecting people all over the country. Why, during 2023, under these conditions, were half a million new immigrants accepted into the already disastrous housing shortage?[26] In another critical observation, it beggars belief that the Australian government is spending billions of dollars assisting other countries to develop their renewable energy capacities, while thousands of families are living in tents in our cities.

Despite our moral and ethical desires for the UN Universal Declaration of Human Rights to apply to all children, women, and men throughout the human family, there is no sign at present that this will happen.

It is obvious that, to paraphrase poet Robert Burns, man's inhumanity to man will continue to make countless thousands mourn.

From childhood traumas to domestic violence, from war to the resulting oppression and deprivation, from famine to the resulting hunger and undernutrition, from natural disasters to the human impacts on the air, land, and waterways, from economic growth to displacement of whole communities, the resulting mental stresses, the loss of personal safety, and the uncertainty of food and water security contribute immensely to poor individual and community health.

When Australian governments eventually took aim at reducing smoking rates through taxation and health warnings, the people responded such that only about 10 percent of the population now smoke.[27] As a result, smoking-related poor health outcomes and associated costs have reduced considerably. It is now time to address the evolving social and health crises as recommended by the parliamentary report on the state of diabetes in the country.

In June 2024, the parliamentary Standing Committee on Health, Aged Care and Sport released its inquiry into the state of diabetes in Australia. These extensive documents involved consultations, submissions from individuals and organisations, time, and a lot of taxpayer money. There are numerous worthy recommendations, including an immediate review of the Australian dietary guidelines.[28]

In addition, there is the Department of Health's National Preventive Health Strategy 2021–2030, an extremely comprehensive 90-page document. It acknowledges that our present healthcare system mainly focuses on treating people who are already unwell. It also recognises that there needs to be collective and comprehensive effort across sectors to better prevent disease and promote environments that support individuals to lead healthy lives. In addition, it recognises that childhood obesity and chronic diseases are priorities and socio-economic status is

strongly associated with health disparities. The document identi-
fies that overweight and obesity are the major contributors to an
array of chronic illnesses, including type 2 diabetes, which impact
every system in the body.[29] The Australian Government allocated
$1.9 million to this strategy.[30] Doesn't seem much when most of
their political announcements talk about projects worth billions!
If their strategy achieves its aims, we shall all be very grateful. My
sceptical self has doubts.

We also have the National Obesity Strategy 2022–2032, which
recognises the extent of the problem of overweight and obesity
in Australia, but also its association with chronic disease.[31] For
example, people who are overweight or obese represent over 50
percent of those with type 2 diabetes, hypertension, and heart
disease, and over 40 percent of those with uterine cancer, gout,
and chronic kidney disease.[32]

The three documents mentioned recognise the relationship
between obesity, diabetes, and chronic diseases and make numerous
recommendations that are similar and relate to ultra-processed
foods, fast food, sugar, and sugary drinks, the advertising of
these unhealthy products – often aimed at children – and their
affordability and excessive availability. A common theme in these
strategies is the need for a greater involvement in prevention. If
the promotion of preventative strategies improves the health span
of the population, it will also lower the risks of developing chronic
diseases. Billions could be saved on primary care, hospitals, aged
care facilities, and pharmaceutical costs to the taxpayer.

Alas, I fear that some national inquiries are for appeasement purposes – diplomatic strategies that may be idealistic rather than acted upon with urgency. Words and recommendations in reports are wasted if not translated into action. Inquiries like the three mentioned allow governments to defer decision-making, allowing them to continue the status quo rather than commit to healthcare reforms that may save millions of dollars in the healthcare budget. By their nature, political parties and governments have many competing interests. I appreciate that prioritisation is influenced by big business lobbyists, local and global industries, international trade and policy agreements, and economics. However, while we patiently wait for the funding and outcomes of inquiry recommendations, the problems of chronic diseases continue to mount up. **This is why your personal awareness of how to achieve good health is so important**. Your efforts to prevent the development of chronic disease cannot wait for the introduction and implementation of the national strategies.

There are many people who wish to focus on their health status, even though there may be no symptoms. They are sometimes referred to as 'the worried well'. The health system promotes early screening for breast and cervical cancer and encourages multiple vaccinations to prevent other diseases. I support the concept of health awareness and preventative care. *So, why not screen early for metabolic dysfunction, the recognised principal factor in the development of chronic diseases?* After nearly 50 years as a doctor, I agree that it will be most beneficial to combine our healthcare system of diagnosis and treatment with a stronger prevention approach. While there will always be a need for conventional and complementary healthcare, you personally can play an important part in protecting yourself from becoming a victim of poor health.

What if greater government action was taken to promote the avoidance of fast food and highly processed foods and penalise fast-food suppliers? For large numbers of people, fast food is all they can afford. It is readily available and convenient. Almost certainly, poor nutrition from fast foods and sweet drinks drives poor health outcomes like obesity and metabolic dysfunction. As the evidence grows that nutrition choices contribute to many of the chronic diseases afflicting our citizens, surely it is time to accept that more can be done. Should commercial entities be held to account by government through taxes for the imbalance inherent in their products between the benefits (affordable, convenient, readily accessible) and the health harms? It is certainly a question worth exploring.

THE INFLUENCE OF THE CORPORATE WORLD

Business has priorities – is your health one of them? Beware of false claims.

Basic fact – the primary function of any business is to maximise the return on investment to their shareholders.

There are many industries and institutions that are directly or indirectly involved in health. They cover food, medications, technologies, universities, government, the medical and fitness industries, marketing, and advocacy groups. The web connecting all these players is extensive.

Let's explore...

According to the authors of a 2022 Monash University study published in *BMJ Global Health,* there is "the increasingly obvious but often ignored problem of the profound influence of commercial and corporate influences on human and planetary health." They call it the elephant in the room.[33]

Let's not forget that the big tobacco companies fought for years against the evidence that smoking caused an array of serious health problems like lung cancer and vascular diseases like heart attacks, stroke, and reduced circulation to legs. They set up research to blame other possible causes for the smoking-related diseases. They blamed consumers for smoking, suggesting they lacked individual responsibility and control. Their enormous financial resources allowed them to use the courts, making it financially difficult for opposers to conduct prosecution. And now they are back in action with e-cigarettes, influencing a new generation of smokers through vaping.

The evidence is strong that sugar is both addictive and has detrimental effects on health. Sugar, its presence often disguised by one of more than 50 alternative names, and its partner in crime high fructose corn syrup, are present in significant quantities in sweet drinks and processed foods. Taking their lessons from big tobacco, the main sugar producers have fought hard to quell concerns. It is on the public record that they paid researchers at a prestigious university to write articles suggesting that the increasing problems of overweight and obesity were due to lack of exercise, not sugar.

Mega-large, processed food companies have global supply chains and the infrastructure and cost of production finesse to swamp our supermarkets with 'foods' made highly desirable through extensive marketing and colourful packaging. These foods require various added chemicals to enhance flavour, resist mould and other infestations, and prolong shelf life. They are low-cost because of the use of cheap ingredients, and sometimes cheap labour, making them affordable foods of choice for low-income families. In some financially deprived areas, they are the only options. For people who are time-poor or have long work commutes, these foods offer convenience. Such foods are referred to as ultra-processed foods, or UPFs. There is emerging evidence that some of these foods promote excessive consumption and addiction.

There have been conferences and numerous scientific articles regarding the possibility that certain foods are addictive. The combination of sugar, salt, and fat from seed oils is often mentioned, a combination commonly present in fast food and ultra-processed foods. It is interesting that sugar and high-glycaemic carbohydrates are the main contributors to addictive traits in human trials. Real food fats have not been shown to elicit behavioural or addictive traits – except in animal models like rats! If addiction is a real outcome of regular ingestion of certain foods, and those foods are also associated with overweight and obesity, the food industry should be challenged. Let's not try the old trick of blaming individual responsibility and self-control.

There are numerous studies suggesting that regular eating of ultra-processed food increases risks of obesity, type 2 diabetes, and cardiovascular diseases in adults. In 2024, the *British Medical Journal* printed articles suggesting the direct relationship between UPFs and 32 different health parameters, including mortality, cancer, and mental, respiratory, cardiovascular, gastrointestinal, and metabolic ill health.[34] Unfortunately, these studies suffer from being epidemiological, and it is difficult to fathom out whether the problem is the sugars, fats, seed oils, the processing methods and extra chemicals involved, or some combination of all factors. Personally, I think that UPFs and fast foods are not conducive to good long-term health.

In some suburbs, however, there is limited access to minimally processed 'real' food (fresh organic fruit and vegetables, free-range eggs, grass-fed beef and dairy, and so on), and affordable, accessible food is found in fast food outlets. Is it the combination of bread and sauces in a burger that is causing poor health outcomes? Possibly. Eating the meat patty, lettuce, and tomatoes is unlikely to be a problem, and so 'nude' burgers may be an option. The universal use of seed oils for deep frying in fast food outlets is likely to be unhealthy, but more evidence is required to substantiate this statement.

Essentially, UPFs may be harmful to most body systems and should be avoided. My own bias tends to accept this probability.

In a previous book, *Our Children, Our Legacy,* I reported on a

2015 *BMJ* investigative feature, 'Sugar: Spinning a Web of Influence', a key feature article that exposed public-health scientists involved with the food companies being blamed for the obesity crisis. These scientists had significant roles in Britain's top two government-funded organisations, the Medical Research Council's Human Nutrition Research Unit at Cambridge and the Scientific Advisory Committee on Nutrition, which between them had received 10 years of funding from Coca-Cola, PepsiCo, Nestlé, WeightWatchers, GlaxoSmithKline, WK Kellogg Institute, Sainsbury's, and Nutrilicious.[35]

In 2017, a study in the *American Journal of Preventative Medicine* highlighted financial sponsorship ties between two major soft drink companies – Coca-Cola and PepsiCo – and 96 US national health organisations. These included the American Medical Association, American Diabetes Association, National Institutes of Health, American College of Cardiology, Institute of Medicine, Harvard Medical School, American Heart Association, and many others.[36] Where is the line between financial support, powerful influence, and hush money?

For anyone with metabolic Red Flag warning signs, or overweight, obesity, or diabetes, consuming sugar will progress them to poorer health outcomes. This applies to at least three quarters of most populations. Must we leave it up to the individual to take personal responsibility and use self-control to avoid these foods and drinks? Or should we look at the political failures that have created social and economic inequities in our population? Should we expect governments to compel Big Food to take its social and health responsibilities more seriously? My advice — don't hold your breath. This is another reason why the best person to look after your present and long-term health is you.

WHO CONTROLS MEDICAL KNOWLEDGE?

This is a serious concern.

Big Food may be adding to worsening health in most countries, but Big Pharma is in another league! Its reach includes governments, drug regulators, universities, institutions, medical journals, doctors, advocacy groups, and you!

Of the 1 million medical articles produced annually, it has been stated that most of this information is unreliable or of uncertain reliability.[37]

Since governments advised universities to connect with industry to gain research funding, most clinical research is about new drugs and medical devices. In many cases, the drug company designs the trials, manages the data, and ghostwrites the journal article. Often, the complete data is not released to the academic authors whose names appear on the article that is then submitted to a medical journal. Indeed, the complete data is not seen by other academics who are relied upon to peer review the proposed article for the journal. Medical journals are financially dependent on pharma money buying thousands of article reprints, which are then distributed to doctors by drug representatives. Doctors, working at the coalface, seem to be unaware of the influence of pharma in this whole process. Drug company junkets for doctors and sponsored meetings are other areas where prescribing habits can be influenced.

Professor Lisa Bero points out, "When big companies fund academic research, the truth often comes last."[38]

Another issue is that authors are expected to reveal conflicts of interest if they have connections to or have received payments from pharmaceutical companies. However, this does not always happen, leaving the reader in the dark regarding the researchers' conflicts and biases.

Of the small number of new drugs that are released in the US every year – that is, drugs that are 'new molecular entities', as opposed to reformulations or patent extensions – only one quarter provide genuine new benefit. The problem is that no one can predict which ones will be useless or cause untoward side effects. There are many instances of drugs being found to be dangerous and subsequently withdrawn years later. In some cases, significant drug side effects were already known to the drug companies, but the information was withheld. Examples abound, for instance, the arthritis drug Vioxx and the opioid crisis that is still playing out in the US.

In the US, the surge of Emergency Use Authorization (EUA) applications and approvals by the Food and Drug Administration (FDA) (one example is the EUA applied to the COVID-19 mRNA vaccines) has helped drug companies gain approvals with less stringent requirements. We were made aware during the COVID vaccine rollout that Western governments negotiated no-indemnity contracts with vaccine providers, despite the fact that the vaccines had no proven short- nor long-term safety.

A major concern is the influence of food and drug companies on political parties and government processes through donations, lobbying, and their role as 'stakeholders' at important policy meetings relating to non-communicable disease (chronic disease) prevention, where their commercial interests are involved. Promotion of their products, some of which have known associations with poor health outcomes, is the goal. According to a 2019 article in the *International Journal of Health and Policy Management*, "It should be widely acknowledged that the current form of multi-stakeholder governance, which includes commercial entities such as alcohol, food and beverage companies as 'stakeholders,' poses a serious risk to progress in the global response to NCDs" (non-communicable diseases).[39]

ENVIRONMENTAL CAMPAIGNS – IN WHOSE INTEREST?

There are many authentic concerns about pollution of air, land, and sea from an overpopulated planet using cars, planes, and plastics created from fossil fuels by big businesses. There is concern that many chemicals have detrimental effects on the planet and human endocrine systems. Herbicides like paraquat have been banned in many countries but not in Australia. It is thought to increase the risk for Parkinson's, a neurodegenerative disease, by a factor of 2 to 6, depending on the level of exposure.[40] There are many more harmful chemicals found in everyday products like cosmetics, toys, pesticides (glyphosate/Roundup), and food and beverage packaging.

It appears to me that many organisations are using global climate change concerns to push agendas that will benefit them rather than benefitting the climate. As I have inferred previously, science is never settled, and although there is a consensus regarding the human contribution to climate change, the voices of high-ranking academic dissenters are being drowned out.

One particular area that I grapple with relates to the use of meat in our diet. You may have noticed that there has been a ramping up in the conversations about the effect of cattle on climate change.

Countries like Ireland are proposing culling thousands of cattle that are being blamed for breathing out such a significant volume of methane gas, influencing greenhouse gas contributions to climate change.[41] The availability of meat, the most nutrient-dense and bioavailable version of the essential macronutrient protein, could be drastically reduced. The latest US dietary guidelines were created by an 'expert' committee that comprised several vegetarian campaigners, and the final guidelines reflected their devaluing of meat in the diet.

The conveners of the forthcoming reassessment of the Australian dietary guidelines have advised that environmental sustainability will be part of their terms of reference. I suspect they will suggest a major reduction in meat consumption.

RANZCOG, my former specialty institution for obstetricians

and gynaecologists, was so pleased to announce the 'special surprise' of a meat-free day during their annual scientific conference in 2023. They are far from the only organisation focused on reducing meat consumption.

In an effort to be environmentally sustainable and reduce the games' carbon footprint, the Paris Olympics committee reduced availability of meat, cheese, and dairy for athletes, and eggs were reported to be in short supply.[42] Athletes know that to obtain complete proteins, animal sources of food are necessary. There was an appropriate outcry.

Then we have C40 Cities. According to their website, "C40 is a global network of mayors of the world's leading cities that are united in action to confront the climate crisis."[43] One of their aims is to have an overall increase in healthy plant-based food consumption, based on the 'planetary health diet', that is, moving our traditional eating away from animal food. There is no evidential support that this major adjustment to our eating pattern will benefit the climate enough to make a difference, and there is no evidence to show that it will not have a detrimental effect on overall health. It is the equivalent of a food-based pharmaceutical adventure into further opportunities for big businesses to satisfy shareholder returns.

Health advice from so many different sides is blatantly biased and encroaches still further into citizens' reasonable choices. We rarely hear condemnation of the food and medication products that are truly of concern to people's health.

Let me remind you that protein and dietary healthy fats are

essential macronutrients for human survival. The best sources of protein come from animal products. Sugared products, and indeed carbohydrates, as a macronutrient class are an option, a choice, but not required for good health. It is possible to be apparently healthy on a purely wholefood vegetarian diet, especially when supervised by a dietician and there is acceptance that some micronutrients may need to be supplemented.

Marketing is utilised by food and drug companies to push their agendas. Marketing for drug products is aimed at you (advising you to go to your doctor if you have certain symptoms), and at your doctor (through drug reps, scientific meetings, and lectures). In fact, marketing accounts for a major percentage of food and drug company expenses. Marketing promotes sales. I recall reading a 1929 statement attributed to a committee of President Herbert Hoover that gave a green light to industry and reflected our consumerist nature, implying that advertising should create "… new wants that will make way endlessly for newer wants, as fast as they are satisfied."[44]

What can you believe, and what should you do? It is no surprise that the public, and probably also the medical community who follow industry-informed government- and academic-sponsored clinical guidelines, are left with total confusion about how to stay in good health. If you wish to take a keen interest in managing your health, my advice is to avoid the big business factory foods and drinks, and eat the best protein and good fat you can afford, be active, recover with good sleep and self-restoration, and foster your friendships and social commitments.

PREVENTION PLAYBOOK
CHAPTER SUMMARY

———————

It is a compromised and conflicted world out there. Without awareness of the influences on health, we become easy targets for those who wish to capitalise on our naivety. You are the best person to plan for your future health.

Chapter 7

RED FLAGS: TRANSITION TO CHRONIC DISEASES

Poor health caused by chronic diseases can take years to evolve. Let's put that into real figures. If you are diagnosed with type 2 diabetes at age 55, your life expectancy will average 6 years shorter than a person without the disease. That would mean death in your mid-70s. In addition, and despite conventional treatment, any or all the blood vessel consequences of diabetes may occur, like vision impairment, cognition impairment and stroke, heart and kidney problems, as well as leg pathologies in nerves, arteries, and skin, and predisposition to infections and amputations. However, it is probable that the real causes of diabetes, insulin resistance and hyperinsulinae-mia, have been actively stressing your body's coping systems from about age 40.

During the interval before a diagnosis of a chronic disease is made, a number of events can forecast future poor health. As mentioned, I call these the '**Red Flags**'. You can consider these as early warnings, the body communicating that all is not well. Occurrence of these alerts should be heeded because they indicate metabolic dysfunction (often with its accomplices systemic chronic inflammation and chronic stress), and so they give you the opportunity to reanalyse all aspects of your health. When Red Flags present, it is time to re-evaluate if you are supporting your body's health needs and protecting it from threats. As already mentioned, chronic poor health often results over time. There are two options: either take the uphill route to restore normal metabolic function or stay on the slippery slope to chronic disease.

The following Red Flags are early warnings, each having the common thread of metabolic dysfunction and, of course, are influenced by the food choices we make.

WEIGHT GAIN IS A RED FLAG FOR METABOLIC DYSFUNCTION

Weight gain can just creep up, and suddenly you know you must do something about it. Weight gain, especially in the abdomen, is one of the markers of metabolic syndrome (that is, insulin resistance and hyperinsulinaemia), a recognised precursor for chronic diseases like type 2 diabetes, heart disease, and cancers. In Australia, 26 percent of children and more than 60 percent of adults are overweight or obese going by the commonly accepted body mass index (BMI) criteria – weight in kilograms divided by the height in metres squared.[1]

BMI, as an index of what represents an underweight, lean, or overweight person, has its critics, so other body ratios are also used to define overweight or obesity. You will notice that waist measurement is important. This is because excessive fat accumulation around the gut, liver, and pancreas is abnormal and represents metabolic dysfunction, often because of overconsumption of certain foods, especially high intake of energy-laden foods, which are converted to fat by the action of insulin.

Ideal Ratios for Optimum Health

Waist circumference. Waist measurement should be less than 80 cm for women and 94 cm for men.

Waist-to-height ratio. Measure both waist and height. Divide height by waist measurement. Ideal is between 0.4 and 0.49. A ratio between 0.5 and 0.59 places you at moderate risk, and 0.6 or more places you at highest risk of diseases related to insulin resistance.

Waist-to-hip ratio. Both measurements are recorded, and the ratio (waist divided by hip in centimetres) cut-off for obesity is 0.85 in women and 0.80 in men.

Body mass index (BMI). Weight divided by height squared (weight / height^2). Healthy weight range is from 18.5 to 24.9.

Extreme weight gain (obesity) has a strong association with subsequent development of all the chronic diseases. The dominant theories as to why you may gain weight or indeed become 'obese' are discussed in the previous chapter.

HYPERTENSION IS A RED FLAG FOR METABOLIC DYSFUNCTION

Let's consider this scenario… You knew you were a bit stressed after negotiating the traffic to and from work, maybe even from the job itself, or you are a victim of the cost-of-living crisis, so you visit the doctor. He or she may notice that your blood pressure is high (hypertension). There may be a prescription on offer, or some tests, and you may be advised to lose some weight and do more exercise. About 1 in 4 Australians have high blood pressure, although for those aged 75 or more, the figure is 4 in 5.[2] Most of these people will be on prescription medications for hypertension.

Until the mid-1940s, high blood pressure was thought to be a normal part of aging. Since then, the significance of high blood pressure and the resulting risk for stroke and cardiac events encouraged the search for causes and cures. Until recently, only around 10 percent of individuals with high blood pressure were found to have a known cause.[3] Since then, insulin resistance and hyperinsulinaemia have been implicated as the major causal factors. High blood pressure is one of the five markers of metabolic syndrome.

And so, please be aware, a diagnosis of hypertension is an early Red Flag warning event. It suggests the need for a metabolic solution.

PRE-DIABETES IS A RED FLAG FOR METABOLIC DYSFUNCTION

Two million Australians have pre-diabetes and are at high risk of developing type 2 diabetes and other disorders related to metabolic dysfunction. Long before a person is diagnosed with type 2 diabetes, the body is desperately compensating for problems related to metabolism, the production of energy, and the use of nutrients from the food we eat. Blood levels between the normal range and the level where type 2 diabetes is diagnosed is a condition called pre-diabetes.

There are no symptoms of pre-diabetes. To find out if you are pre-diabetic, you must undergo metabolic screening through a blood test. This can be part of a routine check-up, but especially it should be performed if you have a family member who has diabetes, or indeed if you are presenting any of the other Red Flags mentioned in this chapter.

Diagnosis of Pre-Diabetes

HbA1c (haemoglobin A1c) between
5.7 percent and 6.5 percent.

Fasting blood glucose between
6.1 and 6.4 mmol/L.

Non-fasting blood glucose level
of 7.8 to 11.0 mmol/L.

The Australian Government and the Australian Diabetes Society have management guidelines for pre-diabetes, for example, weight loss, healthy eating, physical activity, improving sleep, and ceasing smoking.[4] I'll also add stress management to the list, as stress can exacerbate the condition.[5]

Pre-diabetes is a warning. Dietary changes will correct it.

Do not ignore it!

GESTATIONAL DIABETES IS A RED FLAG FOR METABOLIC DYSFUNCTION

The frequency of pregnancy-related diabetes (gestational diabetes) is growing exponentially and is now diagnosed in 1 out of every 5 pregnancies, amounting to 53,900 Australian women affected every year.[6]

Pregnancy has an extraordinary impact on every system in the body. Not only are there psychological and physical adjustments, but there are also major hormonal changes and metabolic adjustments impacting the body's need for homeostasis, the state of keeping everything working within certain tolerable limits. The energy requirements of the woman and the growing baby undergo what must be the greatest physiological changes imaginable. Pregnancy evolves into an insulin-resistant state combined with an adaptive pancreatic response of increased insulin production. The demand for more and more insulin can overwhelm the normal functioning of the maternal pancreas. This is recognised as gestational diabetes.

As a career obstetrician, I saw numerous women whose pregnancies were complicated by gestational diabetes. When I had to contact my patient to advise that her 26-week blood test revealed this diagnosis, I knew that the joys of a normal pregnancy would give way to the anxiety of potential complications. What would this diagnosis mean for the pregnant woman herself, but also for the baby?

Certainly, there are potential consequences for both during the pregnancy, although in general these are managed successfully, including the reasonably common need to have insulin injections. However, it is the longer-term problems that I wish to refer to, because gestational diabetes is an early warning signal that the pregnant woman's body is having difficulty coping with glucose.

For the mother, the metabolic dysfunction that develops as gestational diabetes during pregnancy can persist afterwards. In some women, pre-diabetes may have been present prior to the pregnancy. The risk of developing type 2 diabetes is increased sevenfold over the following 9 years, and tenfold during her lifetime. In addition, hypertension, obesity, abnormal lipid profiles, and various cardiac events are more likely than if gestational diabetes had not occurred. There is also an increased incidence of ovarian, endometrial, and breast cancer in later years. Women who have had gestational diabetes are also at increased risk of developing disabling eye and kidney pathologies.

What about consequences for the baby? Glucose levels that

are high in the mother cross the placenta to the baby. If maternal hyperinsulinaemia is required to control her glucose levels, once her pancreas begins to struggle, hyperglycaemia will occur in both the mother and the baby. Because the placenta acts as a barrier, the mother's insulin does not cross to the baby; therefore, the baby's pancreas must cope with the elevated glucose levels in its own circulation by increasing insulin production. Thus, the baby develops hyperinsulinaemia despite not having insulin resistance. The outcome is a major increase in the risk for type 2 diabetes and obesity during childhood.

The baby brain is especially vulnerable, as 200,000 new brain cells are formed every minute at 20 weeks of gestation. There are significant studies now examining the possibility that a baby's exposure to hyperglycaemia and hyperinsulinaemia during its development causes neuroinflammation, which is associated with ADHD, autism, spectrum disorders, and other potential neuro-cognitive outcomes.[7]

For those women who have had a diagnosis of gestational diabetes, it is recommended that a repeat glucose tolerance test be carried out at 6 to 12 weeks postpartum, and long-term fol-low-up is advised. But who takes on that responsibility? I fear that the follow-up isn't always pursued because of the postnatal demands on the family and the change of medical attendants after the birth. In addition, because the glucose abnormality of gestational diabetes usually 'corrects' itself soon after the birth, the long-term significance can be forgotten. Gestational diabetes is a true indicator of metabolic dysfunction, suggesting a need to focus seriously on taking steps to correct it.

I highly recommend the book *Real Food for Gestational Diabetes* by Lily Nichols. She challenges the Institute of Medicine's methodology for determining macronutrient dietary recommendations for pregnancy, particularly its high carbohydrate recommendation.[8] In a personal communication, Ms Nichols wrote, "Let's turn this diagnosis into a blessing in disguise."

PCOS (POLYCYSTIC OVARY SYNDROME) IS A RED FLAG FOR METABOLIC DYSFUNCTION

PCOS is found in around 10 to 20 percent of women in the reproductive age group.[9] There is a cluster of features including infrequent or absent ovulation, delayed fertility, irregular menstrual cycles, and small cysts on the ovaries recognised with an ultrasound examination. Often, there are other features like acne, obesity, hirsutism (excessive hair on the face and body), skin tags, and dark skin patches called acanthosis nigricans.

As well as delays achieving pregnancy due to infrequent ovulation, there are potential long-term poor health outcomes. These include hypertension, metabolic syndrome, type 2 diabetes, gestational diabetes, and subsequent heart disease and cancer. Ninety-five percent of overweight women diagnosed with PCOS have insulin resistance. Seventy-five percent of normal-weight women with a PCOS diagnosis also experience insulin resistance.

PCOS is a red alert warning of underlying metabolic dysfunction, insulin resistance, compensatory hyperinsulinaemia, and a real potential for chronic poor health to evolve with time.

PENILE ERECTILE DYSFUNCTION (ED) IS A RED FLAG FOR METABOLIC DYSFUNCTION

Wow! Finally, something for the men to worry about. And so they should! It is often an issue so embarrassing that men don't wish to talk about it, and when they finally do, they just want the blue pill. Erectile dysfunction is common, with 40 percent or more of men having difficulty attaining or maintaining an erection.[10] It can start anytime and becomes more prevalent as men age.

There are many possible causes that can contribute to this problem, for example, smoking, drug use and abuse (prescription or illicit), and alcohol abuse. However, ED is yet another early warning feature of insulin resistance, hyperinsulinaemia, and metabolic dysfunction. ED may be associated with one or more of the other metabolic dysfunction conditions such as heart disease, hypertension, diabetes, obesity, anxiety, depression, and other mental health issues.

A thorough discussion and assessment by a doctor will often be followed by medication prescription. However, a reassessment of nutrition choices is vital. Most metabolic dysfunction is caused by insulin resistance, causing compensatory high insulin production by the pancreas. Unfortunately, as you are now aware, chronically elevated insulin levels damage blood vessels, including in the penis, and other poor health outcomes follow in time.

FATTY LIVER DISEASE IS A RED FLAG FOR METABOLIC DYSFUNCTION

Please don't rush past this section about fatty liver because *it is very common in adults and children*!

While fatty liver has been recognised since the mid-1800s, it is only since 1986 that the condition called non-alcoholic fatty liver disease (NAFLD), also known as metabolic dysfunction associated fatty liver disease (MAFLD), came to the world's attention. Now it is estimated that 32 percent of the global population has this disorder.[11] In fact, in Australia, the disorder affects about 30 percent of adults and about 15 percent of overweight and obese school-aged children.[12]

For most, there are no symptoms initially! It is usually picked up with a blood test (elevated liver enzymes) or ultrasound. Often, when they are assessed on a routine blood test, the liver enzymes may be in the upper-normal range. However, normal does not always mean optimal. When I was a medical student, the normal range was much lower than it is now. Left unmanaged, NAFLD is likely to progress to an inflammatory change in the liver called non-alcoholic steatohepatitis (NASH) and later cirrhosis and a risk of liver cancer.

Fatty liver gets its name because of the build-up of a fat called triglyceride in the liver. In concert with the prevailing medical institutions' concern about fats in our diets, it is usually suggested that dietary fats should be removed or reduced. But this ignores the knowledge that it is unhealthy fats from seed and vegetable oils, as well as carbohydrates, especially ultra-processed and refined carbs, sugars, and sweetened drinks, that are converted to triglyceride in the liver.

NAFLD and NASH are the most common reasons for liver transplants. Billions of research dollars have been aimed at finding medications to prevent the disorder from progression – without success. The American Association for Study of Liver Disease (AASLD) has written a management protocol that has failed to stop the upward trends of fatty liver.

The fact is that the disorder is yet another example of metabolic dysfunction, with insulin resistance and hyperinsulinaemia at the core of the problem. Eating healthy fats in a low- or very-low-carbohydrate diet can reverse both NAFLD and NASH, often within a few weeks.

If you are advised that you have a fatty liver, and it is not due to excessive alcohol intake, this is another early warning of impending poor health. Action to improve metabolic function can restore healthy liver function and good health.

EYES – RETINAL CHANGES CAN PREDICT DIABETES, A RED FLAG FOR METABOLIC DYSFUNCTION

I have mentioned that hyperinsulinaemia affects small and large blood vessels throughout the body. It is certain that if your optometrist or ophthalmologist finds blood vessel markings on your retina at the back of your eye, it probably indicates damage from hyperinsulinaemia. This finding may occur years before the recognition of persistent high blood sugars (hyperglycaemia), or the recognition of abnormalities on your tests that would diagnose diabetes. Changes in the retina are significant because they can indicate metabolic dysfunction, and these changes can progress to reduced vision or sudden blindness, or later type 2 diabetes. The occurrence of sudden irreversible blindness is well-recognised as a complication of diabetes.

POOR DENTAL HEALTH CAN BE A RED FLAG FOR METABOLIC DYSFUNCTION

Cavities and tooth decay may be the first warning of poor dietary practices that, if continued, are very likely to result in metabolically related poor health. In Australia, 1 in 3 children has decay in their baby teeth. Tooth decay is Australia's most common preventable chronic childhood condition. In addition, 1 in 3 adults has untreated tooth decay, and a whopping 1 out of 25 have no natural teeth left.[13]

The most likely cause is sugar and sugary drinks, along with frequent snacking and sipping. Ice cream, honey, hard sweets and mints, dried fruits, cakes, chips, and dry cereals are the major culprits, the same that are implicated in the development of metabolic dysfunction and its related chronic diseases.

ELEVATED CORONARY ARTERY CALCIUM SCORE (CACS) IS A RED FLAG FOR METABOLIC DYSFUNCTION

The CAC test is being undertaken by a considerable number of Australians to assess their risk of major adverse cardiac events. A score of zero is desirable because it is proven that a score that's any higher is associated with some calcium accumulation in the important coronary arteries and represents increased risk. I discuss CACS further in chapter 13.

RANDOM BLOOD TESTS MAY IDENTIFY METABOLIC DYSFUNCTION

A general blood test performed for insurance or during an acute illness must always be scrutinised for results that may reveal metabolic or inflammatory dysfunction. It is not okay to accept results that are 'within normal limits'. Optimum results should be in the middle range rather than just within range.

PREVENTION PLAYBOOK
CHAPTER SUMMARY

———————

Recognisable Red Flags predict future poor health. If uncorrected, the inevitable outcome is a chronic disease. Preventative healthcare should include early screening for metabolic function and dysfunction.

Chapter 8

FOOD DECONSTRUCTED

There has been agreement for decades, if not centuries, that nutrition choices have an impact on health and disease. Through trial and error, and scientific research, we know a lot about food being essential for sustenance and, more recently, for enjoyment. We know that consuming too little or too much can have health consequences, and so some people promote the idea of 'moderation' in their food consumption.

Recently, there has been a lot of discussion about the addictive nature of certain food items. In our quest to eat well for health, understanding some basics about food is important.

WHAT IS FOOD?

After the industrial revolution and into the 1900s, better sanitation, treatment of infections and micronutrient deficiencies, and reductions in maternal, perinatal, and childhood deaths allowed researchers to turn their attention to management of chronic diseases, especially diabetes and heart disease. Both of these diseases were becoming more prevalent and were regarded as diseases of westernisation, of affluence, along with gallstones, appendicitis, and diverticular disease. Fats, lack of dietary fibre, and sugar became the research targets.

Research was directed at whether changes in the diet could halt the upward trend in sudden deaths in middle-aged men, along with the terrible consequences of diabetes.

The food constituents that are regularly discussed are fats (particularly saturated fats found mostly in animal foods), sugar, fibre, salt, and seed oils (incorrectly called vegetable oils).

Over time, the diet-heart hypothesis – the idea that dietary fats, particularly saturated fats and cholesterol, cause cardiovascular disease – evolved and gained consensus, initially in the US and later in Australia and Europe, although many eminent scientists dissented. The evidence for the hypothesis was accepted as 'good enough' to make recommendations to the general public (as dietary guidelines). This public policy endorsement gave the guidelines an aura of fact, and they are still promoted today. Indeed, the dietary guidelines have tended to promote plant and plant-based foods, and increasingly advise greater reductions of animal products, particularly meat.

Let's have a quick look at some food terminology…

Basic Food Terminology
(Source: Oxford English Dictionary)

Macronutrients

Macronutrients are the nutrients you consume in the largest amounts. There are three macronutrients: proteins, fats, carbohydrates.

Proteins: Nitrogen compounds, containing chains of amino acids. They are structural (for example, in muscles) and are in enzymes and antibodies.

Fats: Combinations of glycerol and fatty acids. Used for energy, to aid absorption of fat-soluble nutrients and vitamins, and to help provide warmth and protect the body's organs.

Carbohydrates: Sugars, starches, cellulose (fibre). Contain carbon, hydrogen, and oxygen. Used as energy source. Influence blood glucose and insulin levels.

Micronutrients

Nutrients required in smaller amounts: vitamins and minerals.

Organic Food
Living food that has been produced via
farming methods that use only fertilisers and
pesticides derived from natural sources.

NOVA Food Classification
Four grades of processing, from real and
recognisable foods to highly processed or
ultra-processed foods, where there is minimal
real food and numerous added chemicals,
often presented in attractive packaging.[*]

[*] East Carolina University 2021, 'The NOVA Food Classification System', viewed 19 December 2024, https://ecuphysicians.ecu.edu/wp-content/pv-uploads/sites/78/2021/07/NOVA-Classification-Reference-Sheet.pdf.

To recap, food must supply the body with chemicals that will provide for its energy needs and other requirements. Scientists have identified the main constituents of food. There are 3 macronutrients and 29 micronutrients (13 vitamins and 16 minerals). The macronutrients are proteins, fats (also called lipids), both of which are essential requirements in our diets, and carbohydrates. The word 'essential' means the macronutrient contains molecules the body cannot manufacture itself, so they must come from the foods we eat. It may shock you to know that the macronutrient carbohydrate is not an essential food item. Its main molecule, glucose, a useful energy source for all cells, can be made by the liver (gluconeogenesis).

Natural Foods – Traditional Sources

Natural foods come from either animal or plant sources. Animal foods, such as meat, eggs, seafood, and dairy, usually contain protein and fat and very little carbohydrate. Plant foods, such as fruits, vegetables, grains, pulses, and beans, usually contain protein and carbohydrates together. With that said, avocados, nuts, and seeds usually contain all three macronutrients – protein, fat, and carbohydrates. Sugar is 100 percent carbohydrate, and fruit oils and seed or vegetable oils are 100 percent fat.

Ultra-Processed Foods – Factory Made

Ultra-processed foods are highly refined and processed foods and drinks that don't usually follow nature's combinations. Refined food – for example, flour from grain crops – is absorbed rapidly in the stomach, just like sugar. Highly processed foods usually combine carbohydrates with seed oils or other fats, along with added salt and sugar.

We buy food due to its necessity, availability, convenience, and affordability, as well as for cultural or religious needs. Colours, smells, taste, and texture, sauces, spices, and salt can change food from a necessity to a pure pleasure, completely unlike the experiences of our distant ancestors.

But food has changed, and we need to be aware that food production has become a global commercial endeavour, a commodity like gold and oil. It has become more obvious that certain foods and food additives can encourage us to eat far more than is required for sustenance. A big dilemma in nutrition science is the debate around what constitutes the best foods and drinks, and how much the body needs.

In general, you can assume that nature's real foods promote good health, fulfilling your body's requirements for energy and essential macro and micronutrients.

At least 40 percent of food consumed by Australians is ultra-processed and fast food – that is, food altered by factories – and, as we know, 50 percent of Australia's population is living with chronic poor health.[1] Much of poor health is associated with dysfunctional metabolism due to poor nutrition. Some foods are more likely to be associated with the development of overweight, obesity, and type 2 diabetes, which means they are drivers of poor health. Should they carry a black box alert? Maybe even marked with the warning HAZFOOD (my word, meaning hazardous food, like the international warning HAZCHEM, meaning hazardous chemicals)? It certainly seems that way.

MACRONUTRIENTS – PROTEINS

Protein is an essential macronutrient. When food containing proteins is eaten, those proteins are broken down in the gut by digestion to their basic components, amino acids. They then enter the circulation for general distribution throughout the body and are actively absorbed into cells. This process does not require a hormone (like insulin).

Protein cannot be stored in the body, so when protein is ingested in excess of the body's needs, it is excreted, although it can be converted to glucose under certain circumstances. Of the 20 different types of amino acids, 9 are referred to as essential amino acids because your body doesn't have the ability to manufacture them itself. Foods that contain all the essential amino acids are called complete protein foods. Animal and fish sources have all the essential amino acids (and fatty acids), and, in addition, they are in correct proportions and readily absorbed and usable by the body.

There is a hotly disputed situation that becomes significant for vegetarians and vegans. That is, while there is protein in legumes, nuts, and seeds, it is in comparatively low volume and is not as readily usable by our bodies as animal-sourced protein. In addition, vegetables and fruits may not have adequate amounts of the essential amino acids to meet our needs. Some plant foods also contain molecules called antinutrients, which can interfere with the body's ability to metabolise them.

Of course, individuals' food choices may be based on cultural, availability, or affordability reasons rather than worries about adequate protein or its bioavailability. In addition, unlike smaller-scale farming practices, industrial animal farming practices are cruel. Likewise, there are concerns that large-scale single-crop farming practices are destroying the soil and its vital organisms and minerals. What I find more difficult to accept is the drive to drastically reduce animal protein consumption and replace it with plant-based meat substitutes. In my opinion, this is one more push from large food corporations to feed us 'food' laden with chemicals and manufactured with highly industrialised processes. Commerce continually seeks avenues to generate profit, not necessarily health.

Adequate protein intake is important throughout life and particularly as people age. The recommended daily intake of protein suggests a minimum of 0.8 g per kg of body weight per day (a 70 kg person would need about 56 g). But minimum doesn't necessarily mean optimum!

Professor Don Layman from the University of Illinois in the US has spent over 30 years studying protein metabolism. His research shows that, optimally, 1.5 or more g per kg of body weight per day is more appropriate, that is, more like 100 g per day. His opinion is that, ideally, there should be three servings of protein greater than 30 g per meal or 50-plus grams twice per day, with 4- to 5-hour gaps between each meal.[2] Protein volume, time distribution, and quality are important.

MACRONUTRIENTS – FATS

When we think of good health, there is concern about becoming overweight, that is, accumulating too much fat. Additionally, we have been told that fat in our diets (especially saturated fat) will elevate our blood cholesterol levels and consequently our risk for heart disease. We have had over 50 years of government dietary guidelines condemning fat, in particular saturated fat, and food companies have produced many low-fat products. Consequently, when dietary fat is discussed, we tend to assume that the more fat we eat the more likely it is that we may become fat and develop poor health outcomes.

All foods, except table sugar, contain some fat. Cholesterol is a fat and plays important beneficial roles in the body, and the liver can produce all we need if we do not obtain it in our diets. Dietary cholesterol only comes from animal foods. Since the mid-1900s when the discredited diet-cholesterol-heart hypothesis became ingrained in dietary guidelines, dietary fat and cholesterol have been regarded as major contributors to heart disease and premature death.[3]

The fats we consume in food, whether from plant or animal origin, are broken down by digestion to three fatty acids. They are called saturated, monounsaturated, and polyunsaturated fatty acids. They are always present together, although in different proportions.

When digested, dietary fats are either used immediately if needed or stored in our fat tissues. Fat accumulates in our tissues when there is excess fat from the food we eat and, additionally, when fat is formed by the liver via a process called de novo lipogenesis (from the conversion of excess dietary glucose and fructose). Insulin, or rather hyperinsulinaemia, plays a controlling role in promoting fat storage and preventing fatty acid release from fat.

Dietary guidelines suggest the total dietary fat intake should be less than 30 percent of daily calories, and particularly there should be no more than 10 percent saturated fatty acids.[4] Counter to this, some more recent dietary recommendations (low-carb and keto) recommend fat for up to 70 percent of daily calories.

However, as with so much in the nutrition sciences, there are contradictions in the widely accepted heart disease theory that condemns fat. And so, as should be expected from the discipline of science, when a theory is faulty, the hypothesis is wrong, and an alternative is needed. There are now severe criticisms of the research that led to the condemnation of saturated fatty acids, and there are increasing calls for the dietary guidelines to be changed to reflect this knowledge. However, medical dogma prevails long past its use-by date. Hopefully, the authorities will see sense soon.

We need body fat. According to Harvard Health, "Fat helps give your body energy, protects your organs, supports cell growth, keeps cholesterol and blood pressure under control, and helps your body absorb vital nutrients. When you focus too much on cutting out all fat, you can actually deprive your body of what it needs most."[5]

Although there are negative risks if fat accumulates in our muscles, liver, and around the heart or abdominal organs, stored fat becomes beneficial and important under certain conditions. For example, it is normal to have fat accumulation during the first half of pregnancy, because as the pregnancy progresses, the accumulated fat is used to help the pregnant woman's metabolism cope with the energy demands of both her and the rapidly growing baby. Also, whenever glucose and glycogen (stored

glucose) levels run low, the stored fat (triglycerides) is made available as an alternative energy source for the body, pregnant or not.

Fat is essential in our diet. Fat, and its fellow lipid cholesterol,
is involved in the creation of vitamin D, hormones, including the
sex hormones oestrogen, progesterone, and testosterone, bile salts,
cell membranes, and is especially important in the brain. In fact,
the brain has the second highest content of lipids after body fat
stores. Lipids, including fatty acids and cholesterol, are involved
in brain structure and regulation, and make up 50 percent of the
brain's dry weight. Rapidly developing nerve cells during pregnancy and in childhood require a considerable amount of fat for
structure, function, and as a stable, reliable, and efficient energy
source.

Dietary fat is required to allow the body to absorb the vital
and essential fat-soluble vitamins A, D, E, and K. Omega-3 and
omega-6 are two dietary fats that are especially important for
good physical and mental health. They are both essential polyunsaturated fatty acids that we must obtain from the diet, as the body
cannot make them. However, balance is important, and ideally
their levels in the body should be an equal ratio. Some researchers believe that diets high in seed oils unbalance this ratio, with
the amount of omega-6 found to be ten or more times greater
than the level of omega-3. This contributes to inflammation.

So, for the promotion of good health, there is a need for a
reasonable, not a restricted, amount of fat in the diet. But the
type of fat is important. Seed oils (sunflower, safflower, canola
[rapeseed], corn, cottonseed, grapeseed, soybean, rice bran) are

used for cooking and are present in many unhealthy ultra-processed foods and takeaway fast foods. They undergo multiple levels of processing from the seed to the eventual formation of an oil, for example, bleaching and deodorising. Alternatively, oils derived from fruits, like extra-virgin olive, coconut, and avocado oils, have a better balance between omega-3 and omega-6.

MACRONUTRIENTS – CARBOHYDRATES

Carbohydrates are the most abundant macronutrient. They contain sugars like glucose, fructose, galactose, as well as fibre. Carbohydrates are a major component of fruits, vegetables, starchy foods like potatoes, sweetened drinks, and refined (flour), and processed food. When these are consumed, the carbohydrate components are broken down into various sugars, such as glucose, fructose, and galactose, in addition to fibre, which is mostly indigestible. Table sugar (sucrose) is a combination of glucose and fructose. The body is wary of glucose in the circulatory system because of its inflammatory ability. And so, there is a safety mechanism that uses insulin to maintain levels under tight control. Insulin activates cells to absorb glucose. This works well until the cells become resistant to insulin's actions (more later).

Although carbohydrates provide glucose, which provides energy, it is not true that our diets must supply the glucose. If the diet contains an adequate amount of protein and fat, the liver is capable of manufacturing all the glucose required by the body and brain through a process called gluconeogenesis (the new formation of glucose). It is also a misconception that our brains can only rely on glucose as its energy source and therefore we must consume glucose in our diets. Most cells in the body can either use glucose, fatty acids, or ketones to supply their energy.

Glucose produced from digested carbohydrates may be used by cells to produce energy immediately or stored in muscles and the liver as a glucose concentrate called glycogen. Excess glucose is converted to fat (triglycerides) and stored in fat cells. Glycogen stores are used when the post-meal glucose supply runs low, such as overnight while we are sleeping. If we are being threatened, for example, when we run away from a vicious dog, glycogen stores in muscles and the liver are rapidly converted to glucose to supply immediate energy to power our escape. Usually, there is a two-day supply of glucose and glycogen stores.

Glucose is generally the main fuel for vegetarians and people who follow national dietary recommendations that suggest we eat enough carbohydrates to supply 45 to 65 percent of our daily calories.[6] For those people who don't eat plants, the body still maintains glucose levels in the circulation within tight parameters because of its usefulness as a fuel. New glucose is made in the liver from fatty acids or, if necessary, from amino acids.

Carbohydrates also contain fibre from plant cell walls, which, in fact, is not digestible. Fibre is the plant equivalent of bones or skeleton in animals. When carbohydrates are eaten, some foods give up their glucose quickly in the stomach, and this is absorbed into the blood circulation. To prevent the inevitable high glucose spike, fibre is thought to slow that process. Further down in the large gut, fibre is thought to feed the gut microbiome (trillions of bacteria in the large bowel). When the bacteria feed on fibre, they produce gas and reproduce. In just one day, one bacterial cell can result in a trillion new family members, adding to gas production as well as bulk of the faecal residue. Both outcomes can result in bloating and constipation – which is not what we are led to believe. We are also told that soluble fibre reduces the absorption of dietary cholesterol, important if you believe in the discredited diet-cholesterol-heart hypothesis. Unfortunately, soluble fibre may also reduce the absorption of other dietary nutrients.

PREVENTION PLAYBOOK
CHAPTER SUMMARY

———

Food choices have a direct impact on health. Essentially, food is composed of macronutrients (proteins, fats, carbs) and micronutrients (vitamins and minerals). Food choices depend on availability, affordability, accessibility, choice, and addiction. National food guidelines have continued to rely on dietary questionnaires, and exclude many studies about low-carbohydrate eating.

Chapter 9

THE FOOD
DEBATES

Food is an essential requirement for sustenance and the maintenance of life. Like the human body, the chemical make-up
of food is virtually beyond the ability of science to comprehend.
Despite that, the human quest for black-and-white answers to all
things has provoked debates about which foods (and which components of food) optimise and which foods degrade health.

Polarising opinions are debated over and back,
with research usually aimed at supporting strongly
held beliefs rather than challenging them.

The truth may never be found. When you introduce commercial, ideological, environmental, climate, and political influences, opposing sides are taken and 'never the twain shall meet'.

For half a century, dietary guidelines (imported from the US) have suggested that 45 to 65 percent of our daily food consumption should be from carbohydrates (this converts to about 230 to 310 g, which is equivalent to 920 to 1240 kcals). Carbohydrates can be subdivided into simple (sugars) and complex (fibre and starch). Sugars are absorbed rapidly and are likely to cause a spike in blood insulin and glucose levels.

Currently, we have a strong understanding of the role of insulin in health and the development of chronic disease, and the clinical benefit of avoiding hyperinsulinaemia and insulin resistance by reducing carbohydrates, in particular added sugars, in managing type 2 diabetes. This understanding heavily influences my own dietary choices and recommendations.

Let's now look at some of the most contentious debates.

ANIMAL FOOD VS. PLANT FOOD

Firstly, for background regarding the animal vs. plant food debate, I recommend reading a Substack titled *'Harvard Has Been Anti-Meat for 30+ Years – Why?'* from journalist Nina Teicholz.[1] It really sheds some light on the current situation.

Traditional customs and choices in many cultures include animal and plant foods. This combination is referred to as an omnivore diet. However, highly processed and fast foods have changed the dietary landscape.

Animal foods (including fish and crustaceans, beef, lamb, pork, poultry, eggs, and dairy products) are under political and entrepreneurial attack. There are global forces influencing Australia's meat industry, that is, climate activists, animal welfare groups, environment groups, and nutrition groups – or should I say, those who see a potential business opportunity to replace real animal food with fake meat.

Repeatedly, we are told that eating red meat is a less healthy option than plant and plant-based food.

Although epidemiological studies have found an association between meat consumption and a marginal lifetime risk of bowel cancer, this type of research cannot prove causation. The International Agency for Research on Cancer (IARC), an agency within the World Health Organization, issued a 2015 consensus statement declaring that processed meat was a Group 1 carcinogen (a 'certain' cause of cancer) and red meat was a Group 2A carcinogen (a 'probable' cause of cancer). This information was released in a two-page document (monograph) to the world press with no details that independent scientists could evaluate. Even so, the estimated increased risk is less than 1.2 times.[2]

The Australian professor who was lead of the consensus group has subsequently stated that there is need for better communication with regards to their monograph statements. However, a lot of upset and fear was caused by the statements, and there continue to be recommendations to reduce processed and red meat because they may increase the chance of bowel cancer. Yet, while gut inflammation is thought to be the reason for the marginal relationship between red meat consumption and bowel cancer, a 2023 article in the *American Journal of Clinical Nutrition* showed that there is no increase in inflammatory markers in meat eaters, whether the meat is processed or not.[3]

Also, the raising of cattle is stated to be detrimental to the environment by increasing greenhouse gases (methane). Yet there has been a major decrease in the number of grazing cattle and the consumption of meat in Western countries. It is also argued that there is too much land required to grow fodder for cattle when we are facing an increasing world population that needs to be fed. Interestingly, India, the most populated country in the world, where meat is not eaten by the majority of the population, has the greatest number of cattle at over 300 million, in fact 15 times more cattle than in the vast expanse of Australia (2.5 times the land mass of India).

As in other discussions regarding climate, there are alternate views, and I believe it is unlikely that our cattle are 'major' contributors to global emissions. The evidence supporting the contribution of farm animals to global warming is presented in exaggerated terms. In fact, a 2024 report found that the agricultural industry's emissions have been reduced by 78 percent since 2005, much better than the rest of the nation, which hopes to achieve a 42 percent reduction by 2030.[4]

There is no doubt that animal welfare must always be

humane. In Australia, most cattle graze in open pastures, while only 4 percent are in confined feedlots at any one time, where they spend 3 weeks to 3 months receiving grain food and veterinary care.

Those groups advocating meat reduction, or indeed cessation, fail to acknowledge the intimate role of cattle in the carbon cycle, the vital cultural place of meat consumption in Australia, and the vital nutritional role of animal products in human nourishment.

A significant contributor to the anti-red-meat campaign over the last century has been a US religious organisation with powerful allies in the nutrition science world. One of their allies has been the Harvard T.H. Chan School of Public Health, which is responsible for huge long-term epidemiological studies: the Nurses' Health Study 1, the Nurses' Health Study 2, and the Health Professionals Study on male doctors. These studies use health questionnaires that diminish the veracity of the results. Questions concerning vegetarian bias and conflicts of interest have been repeatedly raised regarding their anti-meat campaigns.

Despite these facts, the UN, WHO, WEF (World Economic Forum), and a host of other groups believe that, to protect the environment, we must reduce meat production and consumption, and they are pushing agendas to achieve this. Opportunistic industries developing factory-made plant-based chemical concoctions have been exploiting the opportunity to enhance their commercial interests.

Even Sir David Attenborough, the demigod of planet earth, has lent support. In a personal communication to me, Sir David expressed concern that we may not be capable of feeding the expanding human population because so much land is taken up by cattle and the corn and other crops required to feed them. He also stated that medical studies suggest that if we were to adopt a diet containing significantly less meat, deaths from heart disease, obesity, and some cancers could drop by 20 percent, leading to substantial financial savings. This assumption is completely misinformed.

It is so easy to become swept up in, to comply with, and to blindly accept, political, commercial, and activist ideology and agendas without considering the flaws. It is important to question, to be at least a little sceptical, and to criticise when necessary. But it is becoming less acceptable to do this and avoid being branded a conspiracy theorist or described as pushing misinformation or disinformation. As I have said before, science is never settled (including climate science), and debate and further research will eventually lead closer to the truth.

There may be no answer yet to the posed question – which is better, animal or plant food? Our human selves have eaten animal and real plant foods since ancestral times. Since factory-produced chemically altered foods have recently entered the food chain, there has been an associated rise in metabolic dysfunction. From a personal viewpoint, I have to say two things. I enjoy meat and real plant foods. More importantly, the vital essentials of protein and fat are best provided by animal foods. This is especially true for anybody who has metabolic dysfunction (50-plus percent of the Australian population) and people who suffer from bowel problems, including irritable and inflammatory bowel conditions, because they need to reduce their intake of sugars and processed foods and fibre (carbohydrates).

As discussed, plant foods (carbohydrates) may not be an essential requirement in the human diet, and lowering the percentage of certain carbohydrates (for example, sugars, grains, seed oils, and juices) has had a wonderfully beneficial effect in the management of type 2 diabetes through lowering the need for insulin secretion.

I would encourage strict vegetarians and certainly those who are vegan to seek assistance from a dietician regarding the vegetarian foods and supplements that will give them enough of the essential nutrients and fortified micronutrients for the best chance of avoiding deficiencies that will result in poorer health in the long term.

FATS AND SATURATED FATS IN THE DIET

Prior to the 1950s, half the people who suffered heart attacks died. Management for those who survived consisted of pain relief oxygen and bed rest, and most never returned to work.

Some research suggested that dietary fats, in particular saturated fats, caused heart disease by increasing cholesterol and fatty acids in the bloodstream and in the plaques that narrowed coronary arteries. When President Eisenhower suffered a heart attack in 1955, his physician was influenced by this 'diet-heart hypothesis', and he recommended a low-fat, low-cholesterol diet. In due course, the hypothesis gained favour with the American Heart Association and became a cornerstone of nutrition advice thereafter throughout the world.[5]

While plant and animal foods contain fats, saturated fats are present mostly in animal products. And so, to this day, there are recommendations to reduce or avoid red meats (beef, pork, lamb), processed meats (sausages, salamis), and full-fat dairy (milk, cream, butter, cheese). All of this to keep cholesterol low and reduce the risk of developing heart disease. As a result, we have seen the emergence of low-fat food products, plant-based 'meats', the suggestion to eat lean cuts of meat, and significantly the proliferation of vegetable/seed oils like canola, sunflower oil, and so on.

And of course, medications (statins) are recommended to reduce total and LDL-cholesterol.

But...

Cholesterol has hugely important functions in the body. It forms part of the outer layer (membrane) of all cells in the body; it is needed to make vitamin D and also the hormones that keep your teeth, bones, and muscles healthy, and, very importantly, cholesterol is a significant component in the formation of sex hormones. It is also used to make bile, which is required to help digest fats in your food. The brain produces its own cholesterol because it is so important for healthy brain activity. In fact, 25 percent of the total amount of cholesterol in the body is contained within the brain.[6] In the interest of homeostasis, dietary intake and liver production of cholesterol are balanced – the less fat you eat, the more cholesterol the liver manufactures, and vice versa.

So, are heart associations and government dietary guidelines correct? There is a growing debate questioning the evidence supporting the diet-heart hypothesis, especially given the huge rise in the prevalence of obesity and type 2 diabetes in most countries since its introduction. In fact, since 2010, there have been books, an emergence of previously suppressed trial results from large randomised controlled trials, and review articles that question the evidence for continued recommendations limiting the intake of saturated fats.[7]

Additionally, it is recognised that dairy is the major source of saturated fatty acids in most diets, yet cheese and yoghurt may be protective from coronary vascular disease, and whole-fat dairy may be protective against type 2 diabetes.[8] This suggests that rather than concentrating on saturated fatty acids, other components in these foods may be beneficial (probiotics, proteins like whey and casein, minerals – calcium, magnesium, phosphates, sodium – and phospholipids). In other words, the whole food is more important than the individual chemicals. Likewise, meat is a complex food rather than just saturated fatty acids. For example, meat contains highly bioavailable proteins, iron, minerals, and vitamins.

Many foods rich in saturated fatty acids have other nutrients important for sustenance. Also, the health effects of carbohydrates – like saturated fats – depend on the amount, type, and quality of the carbohydrates consumed, as well as the degree of processing.

Science is never settled. It evolves. You can either choose to accept the recommendations against real animal foods, which have been part of human development for eternity, or explore your options. The role of this book is to try to make some sense of the food debates and recommendations that are circulating today and that are creating such confusion and conflicting advice.

Personally, I avoid ultra-processed foods, seed oils, fake meats, low-fat dairy and cheeses, and I love butter, cheese, yoghurt, and all meats, not just lean cuts.

EAT MORE FIBRE – MYTH OR ESSENTIAL FOR HEALTH?

In the mid-1900s, Denis Burkitt, an Irish doctor working in Africa, noticed that many bowel-related disorders were very uncommon among the local non-European populations – problems such as haemorrhoids, constipation, appendicitis, diverticulosis, inflammatory bowel diseases, polyps in the large bowel, and colorectal cancer. He was aware that the refining processes in Western nations destroyed the fibre content of plant foods during processing, and so he believed that fibre (the indigestible part of carbohydrates) was the magic component that differed between the African and Western diets.

In essence, fibre is a sugar that isn't normally absorbed by humans. However, when for example grains are refined to flour, it is readily absorbed as glucose in the stomach, which may spike blood sugar levels.

Juicing fruit or vegetables extracts the fluid that contains vitamins and minerals but yields little or no fibre. Blending (as in smoothies) is less intense than juicing, and the fibre content is retained.

During digestion, soluble fibre, as in oats, peas, beans, carrots, and apples, forms a gel-like material that passes slowly through the stomach, giving a feeling of fullness, which may reduce overconsumption. It is said to lower cholesterol levels. Insoluble fibre passes to and through the large bowel, promoting a healthy microbiome, increasing stool bulk, creating beneficial ketones (an alternate fuel to glucose and fatty acids), and is said to assist those who have constipation.

A 2017 Cochrane report showed there was no reliable evidence to refute the use of dietary fibre. However, evidence did not support that increased dietary fibre intake reduces the risk of colon cancer.[9]

SUGAR – GOOD OR BAD FOR HEALTH?

The role of sugar in the causation of chronic diseases, particularly type 2 diabetes, has had an interesting history.

Sugar, the granular substance we all know, is made of 50:50 glucose and fructose. Glucose is a common fuel source for the body's cells. In the past, it was assumed that it was a

vital ingredient required in our diet. However, this is at odds
with advice from the Institute of Medicine (presently called the
National Academies of Sciences, Engineering, and Medicine),
a non-profit, non-government organisation of experts and scientists in the US. The organisation has stated that there is no
dietary lower limit to the amount of the macronutrient carbohydrate required by the body as food (that is, you can survive
without carbohydrate/sugar/glucose in your diet). The dietary
guidelines in Australia suggest limiting the intake of foods and
drinks containing added sugars, like confectionery, sugar-sweet-
ened beverages, soft drinks, cordials, fruit drinks, vitamin water,
and energy drinks. In the US, they suggest limiting sugar to 50
g per day, that is, 10 spoonfuls or 14 sugar cubes. Fifty grams of
sugar is about 200 kcals.

When some researchers suggested that sugar played a role in
the cause and progression of type 2 diabetes, the sugar industry
fought back. Even to this day, some diabetes associations suggest
that people living with diabetes would prefer to live eating the
same food as non-diabetics, combined with drugs, including
insulin, that lower blood glucose levels, than to adopt dietary
choices, like very-low-carb or keto, which would exclude their
favourite foods!

When researchers examined the impact of sugar rationing on
pregnant women and their babies (up to 100 days old) in England
during the Second World War, they found that rationing caused
a significant risk reduction relating to the development of type 2
diabetes and hypertension.[10]

Additionally, recent successes with carbohydrate (especially sugar) adjustment has given new hope that not only can type 2 diabetes be put into remission and drugs reduced, but managing the underlying metabolic dysfunction may prevent the disease from forming in the first place. This subject is discussed later.

It can be argued that the concentration on managing blood glucose levels, while important, does not address the central pathology of type 2 diabetes, which is metabolic dysfunction and its associated hyperinsulinaemia. Type 2 diabetes can be prevented or managed by reducing the body's production of insulin.

JUICES AND SHAKES – PROS AND CONS

While all sides agree that food is composed of macronutrients (carbs, proteins, fats) and micronutrients (vitamins and minerals), deeper scientific research has found that some foods appear to have medicinal properties. Popular recommended examples include garlic, turmeric, berries, ginger, green tea, kale, walnuts, and honey. There are so-called bioactive compounds in these foods, such as antioxidants, phenolics, and flavonoids, that are said to have functional traits like anti-inflammation, antibacterial, anti-cancer, or neuroprotective benefits. Nutrition authorities in many countries recommend that fruits and vegetables should be consumed every day for optimum health. Australia has the slogan, "Go for 2 & 5," referring to two serves of fruit and five serves of vegetables per day. For some people, a morning juice or shake can be an easy and convenient way of fulfilling this obligation.

It can be difficult to walk past the fresh juices and shake bars in the large shopping precincts, or the expansive sections in super-markets that sell a range of bottled juices. Exotic colours and names and promises of better health, for example, banishing liver and other organ toxins, boosting the immune system, banishing stress, inducing calmness, and so on, and so on. Enjoyable drinks marketed as health boosters.

There are at least 900 bioactive compounds in plants (phyto-chemicals). While some may prove to be very important, others may have detrimental effects. For example, carotene was shown to have anti-cancer effects. But when carotene was isolated and supplied as a high-dose supplement, it caused an increase in lung cancer in smokers.[11] This questions the belief that supplements of food extracts have benefits greater than the whole food the 'active' chemical comes from.

Juicing extracts the fluid content where most of the beneficial vitamins and minerals are contained, and there is minimal fibre, protein or fat. Fruit juice is rapidly absorbed in the gut. Juice is energy-dense (calories). It contains the sugar fructose, which the body is often compelled to store in fat tissue (see the section regarding Dr Rick Johnson in chapter 10).

Blending, on the other hand, is used to create shakes and smoothies (with yoghurt or milk added), which retain the fluid and also the fibre or pulp, slowing absorption and reducing glucose spikes in the bloodstream and the associated release of insulin.

Food energy is measured in either kilojoules or kcals (4 kJ = 1 kcal). The energy in your juice or shake depends on the volume of liquid. It is common to see people drinking 600 ml drinks, which contain over 2000 kJ (about 500 kcals). This is too much. If, according to official dietary guidelines, the average Australian should consume no more than 300 g of carbs per day − that is, 1200 kcals − one 600 ml juice in the morning, with its 125 g of carbs (500 kcals), would take you almost halfway to the upper limit. Add in the other carb-loaded meals, and the day's calorie and carb count would be massive. These liquid calories add to the risk of becoming overweight.

Typically, people who practise low carb eating aim to have less than 100 g of carbs per day. Many aim much lower if they wish to follow a ketogenic eating pattern, for example, 25 to 30 g per day. If you love to have a refreshing juice in the morning, use only one or two oranges as juice at most, or consider eating the fruit. Remember, many bottled juices may have added sugar and other chemicals or sweeteners as additives.

People who are trying to lose weight, or if they have one of the Red Flag conditions, or have diabetes or fatty liver, should consider avoiding juices and shakes altogether.

CAFFEINE

Like alcohol, caffeine is not a requirement of a healthy functioning body. Yet, it is used daily by most of the Australian population. Caffeine is present in coffee, tea, and chocolate or cocoa drinks, as well as soft drinks, sports drinks, and energy drinks. It is often found in chocolate bars, energy bars, and some cough syrups.

Caffeine is a central nervous system stimulant that is considered to be one of the top-five can't-miss sport supplements. Of course, caffeine products, including tea and coffee, are consumed as refreshing enjoyable drinks, but it may surprise you to know that caffeine also has therapeutic uses in newborn babies whose breathing needs to be stimulated, and can also be useful in managing migraines. Caffeine is said to have several health benefits, including reduction of some cancers, heart diseases, and mortality, Parkinson's disease, possibly Alzheimer's dementia, and type 2 diabetes. However, the jury is still deciding the merits of these claims.

Coffee has become a social and commercial success in Australia, with over 25,000 cafes and coffee shops. As a stimulant, coffee helps overcome fatigue and drowsiness, is (incorrectly) thought to help overcome alcohol-induced hangovers, and when taken an hour before exercise, it is said to increase strength and performance.

The side effects of fast heart rate or palpitations, urinary frequency, trembling hands, sleep disturbance, and feelings of anxiety are dependent on the individual, their body mass, and the dose of caffeine consumed. The side effects are more likely when 300 mg of caffeine is consumed in one sitting. Exacerbation of these effects is virtually universal at 400 mg and higher. Yet, unlike the impact of long-term alcohol, especially on the liver, there seems to be no equivalent effect from caffeine. However, the presence of sleeplessness, anxiety, and so on should suggest reducing caffeine intake.

According to Aroma Coffee Roasters, the amount of caffeine in your cup is dependent on the amount of coffee beans used, the type (robusta beans contain about twice the amount of caffeine as the Australian favourite arabica), how the beans are roasted, and how they are brewed. Allowing for these variables, they suggest the following guideline for determining your caffeine dose...[12]

Caffeine Dose in Coffee

Espresso Coffee

One shot (7 g of beans) = 75 mg of caffeine

Two shots (14 g of beans) = 150 mg of caffeine

In most coffee shops, unless you request otherwise, two shots is the standard in espresso, long black (Americano), and flat whites.

Brewed Coffee

Depends on grind, usually 15 to 25 grams of beans, which is 150 to 350 mg of caffeine.

Food Standards Australia New Zealand recommend a daily upper caffeine limit of 400 mg (about 5 to 6 shots). During pregnancy, 200 mg of caffeine (2 to 3 shots) should be the upper limit, as higher doses have been associated with higher miscarriage rates.[13]

SALT – IS THERE A NEED TO RESTRICT SALT CONSUMPTION?

Salt is composed of sodium and chloride. Sodium is present in large amounts in the body compared to all other electrolytes, and its contribution to the health of an individual is enormous.

Iodised table salt and sea salt have the same amount of sodium and chloride. Iodised salt also contains added iodine, an important molecule for thyroid function. However, most Australians get enough iodine from their consumption of dairy products, cheese, and various seafoods.

For some decades, it has been standard medical advice to limit salt intake to 2,300 mg or less per day, as it has been thought that higher intake is associated with higher blood pressure, itself a major contributor to heart disease. However, science has frequently taught us that attributing chronic diseases to one electrolyte or molecule is too reductionist and simplistic given the wide variety of molecules and micronutrients in food, and the immense complexity of the billions of chemical actions and reactions that occur every minute.

The following are reasons to reconsider salt restriction...

Our present food consumption includes a preponderance of ultra-processed foods, which contain added salt, sugar, and other chemicals. Additionally, insulin resistance, or hyperinsulinaemia, is a common related effect. Hyperinsulinaemia affects the management of fluid balance by the kidneys, involving retention of sodium and other effects that promote hypertension. It was assumed that restricting salt intake would have a beneficial effect on reducing blood pressure. However, this is a marginal benefit of only a few millimetres of mercury (for example, reducing 150/90 to 145/85).

People who adopt low-carbohydrate or ketogenic diets lower their hyperinsulinaemia status very quickly. The kidneys respond and stop the reabsorption of sodium, allowing more to be excreted in urine. This can cause a temporary drop in blood volume and blood pressure, thus creating a feeling of being unwell, called 'keto flu'. When starting a low-carbohydrate or keto diet, it is advised to increase daily salt intake to 1 to 2 teaspoons per day (5 g or 5000 mg).

When you minimise or cease foods that promote hyperinsulinaemia (sugars, starches, ultra-processed foods) and adopt low-carbohydrate or keto eating, it beneficially impacts your blood pressure, and restricting salt is not required.

SEED (VEGETABLE) OILS

I have referred to the negative aspects of seed oils in the previous chapter.

PREVENTION PLAYBOOK
CHAPTER SUMMARY

———————

There are many conflicting theories about the
impact food has on our health. Debates become
polarised and polemic, and the result is confusion.

However...
Our bodies' systems respond well to traditional
foods, supporting my bias towards real food
and the avoidance of foods that contain
simple carbohydrates (bread, pasta, rice), the
avoidance of regular fruit juice drinks, ultra-
processed foods (UPFs), foods that have added
sugar, and foods cooked using seed oils (used
in UPFs, fast food, and home cooking).
For people who have any of the Red Flags, or
blood tests suggesting metabolic dysfunction,
or any of the chronic diseases, severe
carbohydrate restriction should be their goal.

Chapter 10

INSULIN'S VITAL ROLE IN HEALTH AND DISEASE

"The public has a distorted view of
science, because children are taught
in school that science is a collection
of firmly established truths. In fact,
science is not a collection of truths. It is a
continuing exploration of mysteries."
– Freeman Dyson

Those who propose and those who question a hypothesis need equal scrutiny.

When listening to a medical talk, I cringe when I hear a lecturer or so-called 'expert' use the phrase, "We now know..." The implication is that knowledge on that subject is now fact and cannot be contested. But science is rarely settled. All knowledge should be questioned and re-evaluated.

> **"If science can't be questioned, it's not**
> **science anymore; it's propaganda."**
> – Aaron Rodgers

George Bernard Shaw once said, "All progress depends on the unreasonable man," and this, I argue, pertains to nutrition science. The 'reasonable' man accepts without question sometimes flimsy or questionable evidence. This is certainly the case with the outdated diet-heart hypothesis.

As discussed in chapter eight, this hypothesis suggests that cholesterol and dietary fat, especially saturated fats, which are present in higher proportions in animal products, are the main causes of heart diseases. For decades, smoking and sugar were somewhat ignored. And so, to save people from dying prematurely from heart attacks, recommendations in national dietary guidelines suggested lowering fat intake and lowering blood cholesterol levels. Consequently, as animal products are richer in saturated fats, the campaign to reduce meat consumption gained momentum. Food manufacturers created 'low-fat' products, and good and bad carbohydrate intake increased substantially.

Serious flaws and contradictions in the original research pertaining to the diet-heart hypothesis have been identified; thus, the hypothesis should have been dismissed, and alternative causes of chronic disease should have been considered. The continuing support for the diet-heart hypothesis should be scrutinised, as it uses unreliable dietary questionnaire data collection and deduces relative risks of certain disease outcomes from certain foods. Often, the comparison is between animal- and plant-based nutrition. Often, the authors are from one US university. Often, their results receive exaggerated headlines and wide coverage in the media. As a doctor, it has become a frustration to see the diseases of modernity, the chronic diseases of Western civilisation, take hold in most societies, while households do their best to follow the flawed nutrition guidelines around how to be healthy.

The diet-heart hypothesis is jaded. It has had its time but failed to halt the surge of chronic diseases. Change is needed. As allegedly stated by Albert Einstein, "We cannot solve our problems with the same thinking we used to create them."

"From little things big things grow…" This is certainly true in the sciences of health and nutrition. Once it became recognised that chronic non-communicable diseases like heart disease, cancer, diabetes, and dementia are not always separate disease entities but are in fact often clustered together in individuals (multimorbidity due to two of more of these diseases occurring in one person), the common nutrition- and lifestyle-based root causes became headline news. People who develop type 2 diabetes, the banner metabolic dysfunction disease, often have up to five comorbid chronic diseases. And so, metabolism (metabolic function and dysfunction) became recognised as the cause or major contributor to most chronic diseases.

Initially, there were just a few, but now there are numerous researchers, academics, and clinicians, from many different specialties and countries, who understand the contradictions in the diet-heart hypothesis and have explored other possible answers as to why we become prone to chronic diseases. They have been adding to the pool of information that supports the hypothesis that metabolic dysfunction is the common pathology in many diseases.

> **This knowledge will influence how health
> is viewed, highlight how good health can
> be part of a long and healthy life span, and
> explain why chronic poor health does not
> have to be the inevitable lot of mankind.**

The resurgence of low-carbohydrate nutrition as *prevention* is a result of this new approach.

INSULIN – A KEY HORMONE DETERMINING HEALTH

You are probably aware of injectable **insulin**, the injection used by people who have type 1 diabetes. Type 1 diabetes usually occurs in childhood and is due to a devastating deficiency of the pancreas-produced hormone insulin. Injectable insulin was a lifesaver for those children after it became available in 1921. It was many years later before scientists worked out the extensive physiological importance of the insulin produced by the body. Now they know many of its roles and recognise its number one position among hormones. Like so many things in life, there is a safe amount of insulin. Too little – that is, insulin deficiency – will result in type 1 diabetes. Too much insulin, called hyperinsulinaemia, is detrimental to every part and process in the body, and is related to metabolic dysfunction. Often, this will develop into type 2 diabetes and other chronic diseases.

Glucose is a hugely important chemical used by the body. However, it must be kept under control by insulin. Some refer to insulin as the 'master' hormone. Its first function is to keep the glucose level in the blood within the normal range by facilitating its entry into cells. The amount of glucose that enters your circulation is dependent on your choice and volume of carbohydrates (and to a lesser extent protein) and how much and how often you eat and drink during the day. Excessive consumption of sugary and starchy foods or drinks can result in your cells becoming overloaded with glucose, and some resistance to insulin's action may occur (referred to as **insulin resistance**). The pancreas responds by increasing its production and release of more insulin (referred to as **compensatory hyperinsulinaemia**) to force glucose into the cell, or, alternatively, it promotes the formation of fat molecules (called triglycerides).

If the resistance to insulin becomes more intense, the pancreas goes into overdrive and produces ever increasing amounts of this hormone. If this continues in the long term, health deterioration in the form of chronic diseases is inevitable.

Hyperinsulinaemia is an important word to remember. As you shall discover, hyperinsulinaemia causes insulin resistance in various cells and organs of the body. It is associated with mitochondrial and metabolic dysfunction. It causes profound changes in large and small blood vessels throughout the body.

* * *

The following pages introduce a number of heroes who have grappled with the complexities of health and disease, attempting to give us a chance at reducing our risk of developing chronic diseases.

* * *

Dr Malcolm Kendrick – What if Cholesterol and Saturated Fats Are Not the Demons That Cause Heart Disease?

Heart disease is the number one killer throughout the world, although there is competition for that inglorious accolade from other metabolic dysfunction diseases, such as neurodegenerative diseases (for example, Alzheimer's) and cancers.

Attempts to explain the causes of heart disease have centred on the potential roles of dietary saturated fat and the body's cholesterol levels, particularly LDL (low-density lipoprotein) cholesterol. The medical profession has adhered to the concept that saturated fat in the diet raises cholesterol levels in the blood. It is suggested that the cholesterol gets under the internal lining of the coronary arteries that supply the heart muscle, causing fatty streaks and plaques in those arteries. Eventually, the arteries narrow and restrict blood flow to the heart muscle, resulting in heart pain during exertion (angina) or heart attack (myocardial infarction).

Recommendations from national dietary guidelines and specialist medical institutions in most countries emphasise the need to reduce fat intake. This results in increased carbohydrate consumption. Medications called statins, used to lower total and LDL cholesterol blood levels in the hope of reducing the risk of heart attacks, are recommended by cardiologists and their specialist academic leaders for prevention of heart disease (primary prevention), as well as for long-term management after a heart attack (secondary prevention). They are the bestselling drugs on Earth.

As with many recommendations in medicine, there is strong institutional consensus, but there are many dissenters who question the supporting evidence. They point to the contradictions in the diet-heart hypothesis and explain that these mean the hypothesis should be abandoned. Those who propose and those who question a hypothesis need equal scrutiny.

Without doubt, statins decrease total and LDL cholesterol. However, Professor Robert Lustig (endocrinologist, researcher, and author of *Fat Chance* and *Metabolical*) and other researchers explain that there are numerous clinical trials that show that the long-term use of statins for primary prevention of heart disease extends life span by an average of just four days.[1] In addition, every drug has potential side effects that must be weighed against its possible benefits. Recently, side effects like mitochondrial changes, muscle weakness, and type 2 diabetes have been recorded in statin users, which should be considered and questioned before commencing these drugs.[2]

Dr Malcolm Kendrick has studied the causes of heart disease for his entire medical career. Following on from articles and meetings with his colleagues in The International Network of Cholesterol Sceptics (THINCS), he has argued against the obsession with the idea that elevated cholesterol is dangerous for heart health and also against the need to keep it at a very low level in the bloodstream.

Dr Kendrick wrote the 2021 book *The Clot Thickens*, which explores the various theories about the cause of heart attacks. He settles on the probability that many factors can damage the arterial wall, resulting in activation of the clotting system and thrombus (clot) formation at the site, and repair, in turn, leads to plaque build-up. Repeated episodes cause further clotting and plaque build-up and the eventual narrowing of the artery, reducing its oxygen and nutrient supply to the heart muscle.[3]

In a review of Dr Kendrick's hypothesis, Professor Richard

Feinman, a New York professor of biochemistry and medical research, stated, "[Kendrick] provides extensive evidence on the more compelling role of damage to the circulation and the role of thrombus (clotting) and the inhibition of fibrinolysis (clot breakdown)."[4]

In this regard, there is backup to Dr Joseph Kraft's pathological findings of damage caused to blood vessels by hyperinsulinaemia and the associated metabolic dysfunction (which we will discuss soon).

In a similar vein, many doctors, including Dr David Diamond, Dr Aseem Malhotra, and Dr John Abramson, have recorded strong arguments that question the prevailing entrenched diet/cholesterol-heart hypothesis and the demonisation of cholesterol, and confirm its important role in the human body. Their statistical, legal, and risk-benefit analyses of the anti-cholesterol drug management of cardiovascular disease are worth exploring.

Ms Nina Teicholz – Maybe Fat Is Not the Problem

Nina Teicholz is the founder and presently a director in the Nutrition Coalition, a non-profit US organisation. The board of directors and the scientific council have an impressive list of important scientists who are involved in the nutrition space. Ms Teicholz has been critical of the potential conflicts of interest of the committee members charged with developing the US dietary guidelines. She has revealed the restrictions in the committee's terms of reference, which excluded a large number of valid studies showing the benefits of low-carbohydrate nutrition.[5]

Ms Teicholz is a reformed vegetarian of 25 years. In 2014, after 9 years of research, she published an award-winning best-selling book called *The Big Fat Surprise*. The book reveals the weak science yet strong political support for the prevailing dietary guidelines that demonise fats, especially the animal-sourced saturated fats, which are stated to be the cause of cardiovascular disease and heart attacks.[6]

For interested readers, she has published further evidence against the demonisation of saturated fats in the journal article, 'A Short History of Saturated Fat: The Making and Unmaking of a Scientific Consensus' in *Current Opinion in Endocrinology, Diabetes and Obesity*.[7] Ms Teicholz also writes a Substack with fellow author Gary Taubes called 'Unsettled Science', which covers claims made by research articles that pertain to nutrition. Mr Taubes is the author of several books, including *Rethinking Diabetes* (2024).

It is revealing that Nina Teicholz and Gary Taubes, who are non-medical investigative journalists, separately opened the eyes of the medical and nutritional science world to the fact that dietary advice from the US government and medical institutions was severely compromised.

Dr George Cahill – The Need to Guarantee Continuous Supply of Energy... Insulin's Premier Role

In this present era of international reaction to climate change and the drive to 'net zero' by replacing present energy sources with renewable sources, it is an understandable concern that interruptions to the nation's energy supply have become a major issue. Similarly, as I have stated before, human existence depends on a continuous uninterrupted supply of energy in our bodies. This is the case whether we are fed or go hungry.

Dr George Cahill was professor of medicine at Harvard, but he also carried out research at the Joslin Center, the premier diabetes clinic in the US. His research centred around the body's adaptation to fasting and starvation, and this led to understanding the premier role of insulin as the overall controller of fuel mobilisation in humans. Because of his outstanding research, he was invited to give the Banting Memorial Lecture in 1971. His topic was 'Physiology of Insulin in Man'.

In response to a meal, insulin is released rapidly from the pancreas to manage any carbohydrate present. Dr Cahill stated that insulin's principal role is to maintain glucose levels within very narrow limits by facilitating its entry into cells, especially muscle cells. Other processes that can increase blood glucose levels, like conversion of glycogen (stored glucose), new glucose production by the liver (gluconeogenesis), or release of fatty acids from fat, are switched off through insulin's action. Under normal healthy metabolic states, insulin will return to low levels in 2 to 3 hours after a meal.

In the fasted state, there is need for only minimal production of insulin, and its low level allows glucose levels in the blood to be maintained by mobilising stored glucose (glycogen) and producing new glucose (gluconeogenesis) in the liver. In addition, fatty acids can be released for use as a fuel as required, especially if fasting is prolonged more than a couple days.

Another action of insulin is to maintain an optimal storage of glycogen (concentrated glucose) for emergency use as a fuel and, once this quantity has been accumulated, to convert any excess sugar and carbohydrate calories into fat.

During prolonged fasting or starvation, Dr Cahill noted that fatty acids or a lipid metabolite called **ketones** become the body's energy fuel. This is important to preserve brain and mental functions that require a high constant energy supply.[8] And as we shall see, the production of ketones may have a vital role in managing mental health and neurodegenerative diseases like Alzheimer's.

Dr Joseph Kraft – Resistance to the Function of Insulin and Abnormal Elevated Production of Insulin Precedes the Recognition of Type 2 Diabetes

Over several decades, Dr Joseph Kraft performed over 14,000 oral glucose tolerance tests (OGTT) on his patients. The OGTT involves taking a baseline fasting glucose measurement; then 75 to 100 g of glucose is swallowed (equivalent to about two cans of cola), followed by more blood tests at 1, 2, and 3 hours. The OGTT is one of two tests used to determine if an individual has diabetes.

Dr Kraft took further bloods at 4 and 5 hours. The significant additional information that he tested for was the blood insulin levels, measured before the glucose drink and repeated hourly for 5 hours. What he found has immense implications.

Three-quarters of participants had a normal glucose toler-ance result — that is, they were not considered to be diabetic in the defined sense by the medical establishment. However, about 50 percent of those with normal OGTT results had *abnormal insulin responses*.[9] That means they had high and delayed insulin responses to the glucose drink — hyperinsulinaemia. Because some cells had become resistant or intolerant to the effects of normal amounts of insulin (the cells were insulin-resistant), and rather than allowing dangerous high glucose levels in the blood, the pancreas increased its workload to produce more insulin. This compensatory hyperinsulinaemia is the first adaptation after cells become insulin-resistant. Hyperinsulinaemia is an abnormal situation and suggests the body is struggling to cope with the glucose load coming in through food choices.

Dr Kraft was also a pathologist. His legacy to us includes the findings from over 3,000 autopsies he performed. He was aware that animal studies had shown blood vessel changes from hyperinsulinaemia. He confirmed through human autopsies that there was a relationship between hyperinsulinaemia and damage to the inner lining of all arteries and capillaries in the body, large and small. Of special interest was his finding of damage to vessels in the interventricular septum, an area where heart rhythm abnormalities like atrial fibrillation can start.[10]

Dr Kraft was chief of medical pathology and nuclear medicine in a Chicago hospital for about 30 years. His 2008 book, *Diabetes Epidemic & You*, contains an interesting comment regarding whether everyone should be tested for diabetes: "Absolutely not – only those who are concerned about their future."[11] His work has been modified a little by New Zealand academics with whom he subsequently collaborated. One other American research team has also shown the significance of hyperinsulinaemia as a precursor to the eventual development of type 2 diabetes.

The bottom line is that damage occurs in blood vessels all over the body because of hyperinsulinaemia, and this begins many years before blood sugars become abnormal.

Dr Gerald Reaven – Insulin Resistance and Compensatory Hyperinsulinaemia Are Strongly Associated with Many Chronic Health Conditions (Syndrome X)

In another famous Banting lecture in 1988, Dr Gerald Reaven described that while insulin resistance may be a necessary defect in the development of type 2 diabetes, most insulin-resistant patients did not develop diabetes, because the pancreas secreted more and more insulin as required (hyperinsulinaemia) to maintain normal blood glucose levels. Essentially, the body adapts and compensates, potentially for years.

He described that the combination of insulin resistance and high-compensatory insulin was associated with central obesity (around the abdominal organs), elevated blood pressure, inflammation, tendency for clotting, and features of what is called atherogenic dyslipidaemia (elevated triglycerides, lower HDL [high-density lipoprotein], and elevated small-density LDL – later to be called metabolic syndrome).[12] These features, in turn, are related to coronary vascular disease and heart attacks. In addition, the stress-related part of the nervous system, called the sympathetic system, is highly activated (chronic stress response), as are uric acid and kidney retention of sodium. Dr Reaven used the term Syndrome X when giving his lecture, and he was among the first to point out the clustering of these various abnormalities occurring because of insulin resistance and hyperinsulinaemia.

Over the following decades, it became established that insulin resistance eventually causes inflammation, elevated blood pressure, heart disease and stroke, pre-diabetes, type 2 diabetes, gestational diabetes, at least 13 different cancers, polycystic ovarian syndrome (PCOS), neurodegenerative diseases (Alzheimer's disease is sometimes referred to as type 3 diabetes), and metabolic-associated fatty liver disease.

Insulin Resistance Syndrome Becomes Metabolic Syndrome

Reaven's 'Syndrome X' was also called 'insulin resistance syndrome', and more recently, metabolic syndrome, although they are not quite the same entity. Metabolic syndrome is the term used to describe metabolic dysfunction and is diagnosed when at least 3 of 5 features are present (increased central abdominal obesity, elevated blood pressure, high fasting blood glucose, high triglycerides, and low HDL).

Dr Reaven pointed out that although insulin resistance and compensatory hyperinsulinaemia are not the same as metabolic syndrome, they draw attention to the need for thorough investigation of all the features previously mentioned. As I have stated, there are preventative benefits from screening for metabolic dysfunction (metabolic syndrome) at any age in adult life.

Insulin Resistance (Hyperinsulinaemia) Is Carbohydrate Intolerance

In a 2002 article in the journal *Circulation*, Dr Reaven referred to insulin resistance as the body's intolerance of carbohydrates. He clearly objected to using the high-carbohydrate, low-fat diet in insulin-resistant patients.[13] Despite his observations and recommendations, the mainstay recommended dietary advice in all national dietary guidelines around the world, for the whole population, and also for those with diabetes and heart disease, encourages high intake of carbohydrates.

Armed with the knowledge from Dr Reaven, it makes no sense to recommend high-carbohydrate nutrition to people with insulin resistance. Yet Diabetes Australia suggests there is no special diet needed for those with diabetes, and they can eat the same foods as everyone else.[14]

Dr Rick Johnson – Fructose... Does It Contribute to Insulin Resistance?

So far in this book, I have emphasised that insulin resistance and compensatory high blood insulin (hyperinsulinaemia) cause disruption of normal metabolic function. I have explained that the conventional medical approach delays diagnosis of metabolic dysfunction until features related to metabolic syndrome are found or when a chronic disease is diagnosed, such as type 2 diabetes, or cardiovascular complications. Dr Rick Johnson believes that fructose may be a primary cause of cells reducing their sensitivity to the effects of insulin – that is, insulin resistance – and may be a major trigger for obesity development.[15]

Dr Johnson is a professor of medicine and researcher at the University of Colorado. As a kidney specialist, he has seen the devastating destruction of kidney function related to obesity and type 2 diabetes. It is acknowledged that most people who must undertake kidney dialysis have diabetes.

Dr Johnson has spent years piecing together why *fructose* plays a significant role in fuelling obesity. His research has culminated in lectures, videos, and a 2022 book called *Nature Wants Us to Be Fat*. He and his team of researchers have hypothesised that humans have a fructose-powered 'survival switch', a metabolic pathway that turns fat storage on and off.[16] In our distant past, famine was not uncommon, and this switch played an important role in our survival. In the animal world, the survival switch explains the fat accumulation that occurs before hibernation. Dr Johnson's research suggests that the modern human diet has permanently fixed the survival switch in the 'on' position, leading to metabolic dysfunction, obesity, and the other chronic diseases responsible for poor health and premature death.

Fructose is one half of sucrose (table sugar). The other half is glucose. Fructose is the dominant 'sugar' in fruit. Fructose gives sugar its sweetness. It is not merely the fructose we eat that causes obesity; it is the fructose the body makes as well. Dietary fructose comes from sugar, sugary drinks (which often contain high fructose corn syrup), and alcohol (especially beer). Unfortunately, alcohol acts like a sugar! The body produces fructose when we eat high-glycaemic and salty foods. Soft drinks not only provide fructose, but can also triple the production of fructose within the body.

Dr Johnson believes that fructose (ingested and fructose man-ufactured in the body) is a cause of insulin resistance, leading to hyperinsulinaemia, metabolic dysfunction, and subsequent fat storage.

Dr Sarah Hallberg – Management of Metabolic Dysfunction Requires Lowering Hyperinsulinaemia by Reducing Certain Carbohydrates

In 2019, I had the honour of attending a lecture given by Dr Sarah Hallberg at a Low Carb conference in Denver, Colorado. I can still remember this vivacious woman already engaging the audience as she walked across the presentation platform. "We have the answer," she repeated. She was referring to the results of a large study that she directed with Virta Health at Indiana University that showed diabetes reversal through low-carb nutrition, reducing, or even reversing, the need for diabetes medications or weight loss surgery.[17]

In 2015, as adjunct professor of medicine at the University of Indiana and founder of their obesity clinic, Dr Sarah stunned the diabetes and nutrition world with her TEDx Talk presentation titled 'Reversing Type 2 Diabetes Starts with Ignoring the Guidelines', which has been viewed around 11 million times on YouTube. Recognising that refined foods, refined sugars, and processed foods are related to the development of overweight, obesity, and type 2 diabetes, she instituted a low-carbohydrate program for her patients with great success.[18]

Dr Sarah worked with remarkable low-carb researchers like Jeff Volek, Stephen Phinney, and a large team at Virta Health in the US, who have done so much to give hope to people with metabolic dysfunctions like obesity and type 2 diabetes. In 2022, Virta's 5-year data showed sustained blood sugar control, medical deprescription, weight loss, and improved cardiometabolic markers like HDL, triglycerides, and inflammation.[19] These outcomes are particularly encouraging, as type 2 diabetes was previously considered a progressive disease, even when treated with medications.

Dr Sarah, a non-smoker, died from metastatic lung cancer in 2022 at age 50. She remains an inspirational hero whose one goal was to give hope to the many who suffer with chronic disease.

Dr David Unwin – Translating the Low-Carb Science into Clinical Use

In the last decade, several researchers and individual doctors, including Dr David Unwin from the UK, noticed dramatic improvement after offering patients living with type 2 diabetes either a trial of dietary changes or conventional medical treatment. By cutting out sugar as well as highly processed and refined foods and drinks, and with further reductions in high-glucose-load vegetables and fruits (no need to count calories), he was thrilled to report a 51 percent diabetes remission rate in the diet change group.[20]

Dr Unwin has contributed several highly respected articles to medical journals, based on his clinical findings gained in the real-life setting of general practice. He has also produced colourful, freely available sugar infographics that practitioners and people with diabetes, indeed anyone, can access to guide their dietary choices.

In 2018, as the tide was turning, there were – perhaps reluctant – publications from the US, UK, and EU accepting low-carbohydrate management of diabetes. Now the dietary management recommendations include very-low-carbohydrate nutrition. Dr Unwin and many others have assisted thousands of individuals with type 2 diabetes to reduce or cease their medications while keeping the disease in remission.

Dr Jason Fung – Intermittent Fasting

Dr Jason Fung is a Canadian kidney and obesity specialist. With over a decade of experience helping his obese and diabetic patients with kidney diseases lose weight, he is considered one of the leading exponents of the benefits of intermittent fasting, drawing on research from George Cahill, who quantified the body's response to fasting and starvation. He and his work partner, Megan Ramos, have thousands of delighted clients who have lost weight and changed their lives permanently.

Dr Fung has several best-selling books. *The Obesity Code* and *The Complete Guide to Fasting* are informative and easy to digest (pun).

Dr Peter Brukner – Defeat Diabetes

Dr Peter Brukner, an Australian professor of sports medicine, is a former team doctor for topflight cricket and soccer teams, author of sports medicine textbooks, and now founder of Defeat Diabetes, a national company that has been helping Australians put their type 2 diabetes into remission. Dr Peter himself was a victim of the Red Flag metabolic dysfunction conditions of obesity and fatty liver. He corrected these through eating a low-carb healthy-fat diet (LCHF).

Diabetes Australia has joined forces with Defeat Diabetes to reach out to Australia's 1.3 million diabetics, with a combined goal of achieving type 2 diabetes remission in 100,000 Australians.[21] This is an extraordinary development showcasing the acceptance of the strong evidence for sugar and carbohydrate restriction in the management of patients suffering from type 2 diabetes.

Professor Bruckner has a superb associate, Dr Paul Mason. Dr Mason's educational videos are outstanding, and I highly recommend them. As an aside, he can do more chin-ups than most personal trainers!

Dr Rod Tayler and Dr Jeffry Gerber – Bringing Low-Carb to the World

Dr Rod Tayler, an anaesthetist in Melbourne, and Dr Jeffry Gerber, an MD in Denver, Colorado, met at a ski resort several years ago. Sharing a similar deep interest in the role of nutrition for good health, and the slowly evolving advice around alternative nutrition, resulted in low-carb conferences in Australia and the US. Their conferences and lecture videos attract massive attention in numerous countries.

They and their network of enthusiastic evidence-based presenters are significant contributors to the groundswell movement promoting health through better nutrition. YouTube videos of their conferences are free and a great place to start your personal journey of considering better nutrition for your health before medications.

DIGGING TO THE TRUTH

I understand how confusing it can be when your goal is to do your best for yourself, your family, and your society. When we wash away the biases and marketing, I believe we have reached a state of knowledge that seems to be getting closer to the truth of how best to support our bodies to gain good health.

The heroes I have discussed have made important advances in our pool of knowledge. It is not unexpected that biased groups and individuals will try to maintain the failed health advice. But the evidence is now supporting the new science of health and the importance of metabolic function.

**PREVENTION PLAYBOOK
CHAPTER SUMMARY**

Insulin is the master hormone promoting healthy metabolism and normal health but also contributes to metabolic dysfunction and chronic diseases. To control health, you must control metabolism and the hormone insulin.

"Reversing type 2
diabetes starts with
ignoring the guidelines."

– Dr Sarah Hallberg

Chapter 11

LESSONS FROM TYPE 2 DIABETES – REVERSAL AND PREVENTION

A common chronic disease present in 1 in 20 Australians and has devastating effects on sufferers' health can now be put into remission through dietary changes. For more than 50 percent of people living with type 2 diabetes, medications can be ceased, and blood test results can be returned to normal.

This is OUTSTANDING news.

The type 2 diabetes success story has given new hope to patients and doctors alike. However, only small numbers of sufferers are aware of the news.

It is worthwhile further discussing type 2 diabetes, the poster child of metabolic dysfunction. It serves as an interesting case study that will give us direction as to how to prevent the poor health it causes and indeed how to reduce your risk of being diagnosed with it or other metabolic disorders. There are different subtypes of diabetes. In this section, I am referring to the most common form, type 2 diabetes.

THE DIABETES STORY

Diabetes is the epitome of metabolic dysfunction. Type 2 diabetes is at epidemic prevalence in the world. As mentioned, 1 in 20 Australians are living with diabetes, representing an almost tripling in incidence from 2000 to 2021.[1]

> **Among chronic diseases, diabetes is in the top ten; however, it is also associated with nearly all of the other chronic diseases that cause long-term illness and premature death.**

For example, individuals whose cause of death is recorded as diabetes often also have 5 to 6 associated chronic diseases, suggesting that they may have similar causation, namely metabolic dysfunction. Individuals living with diabetes often have hypertension, coronary heart disease, fatty liver disease, neurode-generative disorders and/or chronic kidney disease.

Type 2 diabetes is diagnosed by your doctor when a blood test (oral glucose tolerance test [OGTT]) reveals high glucose levels in your blood, or with a different blood test called HbA1c. Through these tests, we have learnt that 1.3 million Australians live with diabetes and another 2 million have pre-diabetes.[2] In addition, it is estimated that another 500,000 have type 2 diabetes but haven't been tested yet (taken together, this represents 1 in 7 people!).[3]

The major concern about a new diagnosis of type 2 diabetes is that the disease has already been brewing for maybe 10 or 15 years! Even the major medical institutions recognise terms like pre-diabetes and impaired glucose tolerance. These are manifestations of metabolic dysfunction and are accompanied for years by destructive hyperinsulinaemia. Hyperglycaemia (persistently raised blood glucose levels) is the medical hallmark of diabetes, but it is a very late manifestation after years of worsening metabolic function.

A big issue is that the medical profession and their academic leadership have paid more attention to the late occurrence of high blood sugar levels (hyperglycaemia); meanwhile, for several years, hyperinsulinaemia will have created mayhem throughout the body.

Historically, diabetes has been recognised since 1500 BC and was named in about 250 BC. The role of the pancreas was recognised in 1889. In 1910, a secretion from the pancreas (named insulin) was shown to control glucose metabolism. Insulin was isolated in 1921 in Canada by Banting and Best and was used as treatment soon after. In 1936, Sir Harold Himsworth distinguished the difference between type 1 (insulin deficiency) and type 2 (insulin resistance). In type 2, large increases of insulin (hyperinsulinaemia) are required to maintain normal glucose levels in the circulation by disposing of it into cells. Eventually, the pancreas struggles to produce such high levels of insulin, and glucose levels in the circulation rise (hyperglycaemia), resulting in symptoms that lead to medical attention and diagnosis of type 2 diabetes.

Prior to 1920, fasting or low-carbohydrate diets were used to manage diabetes, and medically supervised ketogenic diets (very low or no carbohydrates) were used to treat intractable epilepsy. After the development of insulin injections and subsequently blood-sugar-lowering medications, the dietary approach to treatment was relegated to the background.

Many people with type 2 diabetes do not experience symptoms, and the condition may be present for years before diagnosis (that is, pre-diabetes). Unfortunately, slow but progressive damage happens before the eventual diagnosis due to the vascular effects of hyperinsulinaemia as shown by Dr Kraft. The usual management is drugs, diet, and exercise, and, despite medications, diagnosed individuals are told that diabetes is a progressive and

lifelong disease. Clinical outcomes include the long-term consequences of blindness, amputations, kidney failure, heart attacks,
and dementia, and diabetics die on average 6 years earlier than
non-diabetics, despite treatment.[4]

WHY ARE WE CHOOSING SUPPRESSION OVER REMISSION?

First-line pharmaceuticals – that is, the preferred medications for
treating diabetes – at lowest doses have only short-term benefits
on blood sugar responses and often require increased dosage and
the addition of second- or third-line medications, and finally
insulin injections.

Prevailing recommended dietary advice from the Australian
Dietary Guidelines and an attitude that people with diabetes
should be able to eat the same foods as the rest of the family
seems totally illogical. On the Diabetes Australia website is the
following statement: "There is no such thing as a diabetic diet.
People living with diabetes can enjoy the same foods as everybody
else."[5] The nutrition that resulted in the disease in the first place
is recommended. Is this advice given because they believe that
regardless of blood glucose levels caused by food, the medications
will bring them down? Is this the reason why diabetes experts
have stated that the disease is a lifelong progressive disease? I am
dismayed that doctors and dieticians are told to recommend the
prevailing guidelines.

The critical takeaway from the findings of Cahill, Kraft,

Reaven, Hallberg, Unwin, and others is that type 2 diabetes is a problem of carbohydrate intolerance (especially sugar and starches in all forms), creating a pancreatic response (hyperinsulinaemia), initially physiological and adaptive, but subsequently pathological and destructive. Now, gratefully, low-carbohydrate and keto diets are putting type 2 diabetes into remission, and often meds can be reduced or ceased.

IT IS TIME TO TAKE CONTROL OF DIABETES

Obesity often accompanies type 2 diabetes. Obesity treatments – such as bariatric surgery, very-low-calorie diets, and recently anti-obesity medications like semaglutide (Ozempic) – are also successfully improving outcomes for those living with type 2 diabetes.

The logical and exciting probability is:

Any metabolic disorder that can be managed by nutrition adjustment raises the exciting probability that a similar dietary approach may enhance good health outcomes and prevent the development of metabolic dysfunction and resulting chronic diseases.

Until recently, type 2 diabetes was considered a chronic, progressive, debilitating illness that eventually causes an extensive

array of troublesome effects on eyes including sudden blindness, damage to the heart, brain, kidneys, liver, blood vessels of
nerves and skin, as well as significantly shortening life expectancy,
despite medications. In addition, type 2 diabetes is a major associated factor with most of the other non-communicable chronic
diseases.

In Australia, the UK, and USA, thousands have benefitted
from a simple dietary change because it addresses the root causes
of type 2 diabetes. This success story has been an inconven-
ient outcome for food and pharmaceutical companies. Diabetes
organisations in Europe, the US, and Australia rather reluc-
tantly admitted that the disease could be put into remission,
often without the need for drugs. This has exposed the possibility that pharmaceutical management of chronic diseases does
not have to be the first option for those who are given a new
diagnosis.

The healthcare systems and budgets in Australia and many
other countries are buckling because of the worsening health of
their populations. The present system is reactive, concentrating
more on remediation of diagnosed disease rather than prevention. This has been recognised in the House of Representatives
Standing Committee's 2024 'Inquiry into Diabetes.' Not only
is diabetes a present and future concern, but there is also an
ever-worsening trend in the incidence of other chronic diseases.[6]

Once considered to be the inevitable consequence of aging,
tragically many chronic diseases are being diagnosed in younger
age groups. Obesity (yes, it should be considered a disease),

212 MAKING SENSE OF HEALTH

heart disease, cancers, fatty liver disease, diabetes, chronic kidney disease, mental health disorders, and neurodegenerative diseases like Alzheimer's dementia (often referred to as type 3 diabetes) create years of morbidity. There becomes a dependence on the healthcare system, and frequently these diseases result in premature death, that is, before the age of 75.

While there may be more than one contributing factor to the development of the various chronic diseases, it has become increasingly obvious that metabolic dysfunction, along with chronic stress and systemic chronic inflammation are either the root causes or major contributors. Almost 90 percent of the United States population have abnormal metabolism predisposing them to all chronic diseases, and Australia, New Zealand, and European countries are trending the same way. Despite trillions of dollars being spent on healthcare clinically and on research, there seems to be no improvement at national levels.

Gratefully, science continues to evolve. Gradually, deeper knowledge about the amazing physiological processes and the essential needs of the human body are being understood. In addition, there is a refocus on the pathological determinants of chronic diseases, with renewed attention being paid to the related roles of metabolic health, chronic stress, and inflammation. These scientific advances are challenging long-held beliefs regarding health and disease and are slowly entering the very confused public and institutional health literature. In addition, governments understand the socio-economic determinants of chronic disease, but political action remains in the slow lane.

You do not need a medical degree or PhD to understand the drivers and determinants of health and disease. With this book, I am highlighting the knowledge you need to support normal body processes and avoid or reduce the factors that degrade your health.

Your health is yours to control. Become informed and take action.

PREVENTION PLAYBOOK
CHAPTER SUMMARY

If established type 2 diabetes can be reversed with dietary changes, surely it can be prevented by using the same dietary change. In addition, because the pathology of most chronic diseases has the same contributing pathways as type 2 diabetes, there is hope that a similar dietary approach will aid prevention or remission of these diseases. More and more, this is proving to be true.

"Whenever I meditate on a disease, I never think of finding a remedy for it, but rather a means of preventing it."

– Louis Pasteur

Chapter 12

NEW HOPE TO PREVENT AND TREAT OTHER CHRONIC DISEASES

**Mental health
Neurodegenerative diseases
Cancer**

MENTAL HEALTH – COULD METABOLIC DYSFUNCTION BE THE PRIMARY PATHOLOGY?

Should mental health specialists recommend nutrition therapy?

About 3 million Australians (1 out of 7 people) and about 40 million in the US take antidepressants, and mental health disorders are reported by 20 percent of Australians.[1] The significant increases of anxiety, depression, ADHD, bipolar, and schizophrenia are impacting all age groups. There are numerous triggers that can result in long-term mental health issues, for example, childhood trauma, postnatal depression, and substance abuse. Problems have been exacerbated by COVID lockdowns, personal safety concerns, housing, financial problems, and more.

As a background, since the 1980s, chemical imbalances, particularly serotonin and dopamine, have been promoted as the primary pathology for psychiatric conditions, especially depression. Many mental health pharmaceutical drugs, like Pfizer's Zoloft, are prescribed to correct these alleged imbalances. Frontline doctors will attest to improvements in response to anti-anxiety medication, antidepressants, and other pharmaceuticals. Individuals who suffer from psychiatric conditions can experience life-changing benefits.

Unfortunately, however, as with any medication, derived benefits may come with unacceptable side effects. Some cause weight gain, loss of sex drive, sleepiness or, its opposite, difficulty sleeping, and even suicidal ideation. Medication withdrawal can be problematic for the patient.

For many years, articles have questioned the overall benefits of antidepressant drugs compared with placebo. In addition, the whole idea of a chemical imbalance causing mental disease has been criticised, as there is no supportive evidence, and no reliable blood marker of mental illness has been found. Even as early as 1997, Irish psychiatrist and author Dr David Healy, in his book *The Antidepressant Era*, noted the lack of evidence supporting the chemical imbalance theory.[2] While there may be some disturbance in the balance between neurotransmitters, abnormalities in metabolism in the brain can lead to insulin resistance, chronic inflammation, and oxidative stress (all components of metabolic dysfunction). This brings us back to the possibility that food and its metabolism may have a major role in brain health.

Fortunate clinical observations have influenced science numerous times in the past. For example, there is a fascinating story from psychiatrist Dr Chris Palmer. One of his long-term patients who was being treated for a serious mental affliction called schizoaffective disorder was gaining a lot of body weight. Dr Palmer was aware of keto diets being successfully used for the brain problem of intractable epilepsy and advised his patient to try keto nutrition (very-low-carbohydrate diet). The patient noticed improvements in weight, but also in his mental state, such that by four months he felt 'normal'. After extensive research, Dr Palmer suggested keto diets to others with serious mental health issues. After many more successes, he wrote the compelling book *Brain Energy*.[3]

In 2024, psychiatrist Dr Georgia Ede wrote a comprehensive yet very readable book, *Change Your Diet, Change Your Mind*, affirming her own research and her patients' successes with dietary adjustment to improve metabolic function in their brains.

Dr Ede herself was eating the recommended nutrition as suggested by the US dietary guidelines, leading to the development of migraines, fatigue, body aches, and stomach pain in her 40s. With no diagnosis or successful treatment from the doctors she consulted, she began to experiment with her diet and found that a mostly meat diet made her feel better than she ever had before.

> **Despite being a medical specialist already, Dr Ede undertook a nutrition graduate course at Harvard and realised that nearly everything she thought she knew about nutrition was wrong.**

There was no science behind the official recommendations that had wreaked havoc on her health.[4]

Both books (*Brain Energy* and *Change Your Diet, Change Your Mind*) and an earlier book called *Grain Brain* by Dr David Perlmutter drew attention to the significant influence of food choices on mental health, and on the importance of energy use by the brain. As previously stated, while weighing only 2 percent of your bodyweight, your brain uses 20 percent of the energy you produce. Mitochondria in every part of the body function best when offered good nutrition.

The very-low-carbohydrate and keto diets have found a place in neurology, treating epilepsy, multiple sclerosis, Parkinson's disease, migraine headaches, and vertigo. Why not in mental health disorders too? In the presence of insulin resistance, glucose use by brain cells for energy becomes less efficient. The keto diet creates an alternative fuel for brain cells in the form of ketone bodies, made from fatty acids by the liver. Ketone bodies can cross the blood-brain barrier, overcoming the brain cells' reliance on glucose.

There are now multiple centres and psychiatric institutions researching the potential to use nutrition as a primary or adjunctive treatment option for mental health disorders. This is exciting news, and nutrition could also assist in the treatment of neurodegenerative disorders.

NEURODEGENERATIVE DISORDERS – COULD METABOLIC DYSFUNCTION BE THE PRIMARY PATHOLOGY?

Alzheimer's disease, sometimes referred to as type 3 diabetes, is the commonest neurodegenerative disease and imposes a shocking future for those who are diagnosed with it. It is estimated that around 10 percent of Australians over the age of 65 have dementia, and the majority are women.[5] The disease takes a long time to show the recognisable features like memory loss, meaning that the diagnosis is usually late in the progression of the disease. Money and research aimed at medication treatments have not resulted in highly successful drugs.

But research showing a link between insulin resistance and brain function shows that in the presence of elevated blood and brain sugar levels, insulin is obstructed from crossing the blood-brain barrier.[6] So, there are high levels of glucose in the brain but minimal insulin to get it into brain cells. With reduced energy available, brain cells start to die off.

Ketogenic diets may offer hope, as fatty acids are made into ketone bodies, which can cross the blood-brain barrier and thus become a source of brain cell energy. Prevention is a real hope for us all if we adopt nutrition that reduces the need for an insulin response, and in turn promotes good brain and body metabolic function.

CANCER – GENETIC DISEASE? CONSEQUENCE OF METABOLIC DYSFUNCTION? OR BOTH?

Should cancer teams recommend nutrition therapy?

Receiving a cancer diagnosis is probably the greatest health fear that most people have. Unfortunately, if a cancer begins to spread around the body, treatment with surgery, radiation, or chemotherapy is likely to fail. Recently, the introduction of medications called immune therapies have shown new promise. Unfortunately, cancer cells are like bacteria, and they can become resistant to treatment quickly, and the disease can relapse.

Genetic Theory of Cancer

The possibility that cancer is a genetic disease has dominated research and treatment investigations since the 1970s. However, there is no genetic screen for cancer as such, although there are useful chemical markers. Also, no one single gene has been shown to mutate across all cancers. There are 1,000 cancer-associated genes, some known to promote cancer, and others known to suppress normal genetic activity. Another problem is that the number of gene mutations in a cancer increases as tumour cells progress into advanced stages.

Metabolic Theory of Cancer

Prior to the *genetic theory of cancer*, it was thought that cancer may be a metabolic problem, and this idea has resurfaced over the last number of years. According to the CDC, **obesity** is associated with at least 13 of the known 200 different cancers. For example, meningioma (brain), oesophagus, stomach, pancreas, gallbladder, colon and rectum, liver, kidney, thyroid, breast, uterus, ovary, and a blood cancer called multiple myeloma.[7]

You may be aware that PET (positron emission tomography) scans are used to identify cancer or metastatic cancer no matter which cancer type is being investigated. This takes advantage of the knowledge that the growth of cancer requires a lot of energy (glucose) to fuel its expansion and growth. It has also been shown that another dietary product, glutamine, is required in large quantities. Glutamine is the most abundant amino acid (protein) in your body. Protein production is a function that demands high energy. This is another reason to think there is a major metabolic shift in the development of cancer.

SO, WHICH THEORY IS CORRECT?

There is still great scientific debate as to whether cancer is genetic or due to metabolic dysfunction, or some combination of both. Does a metabolic abnormality create genetic mutations, or vice versa? It is now accepted in many cancer treatment facilities to recommend dietary glucose restriction, for example, ketogenic diet, as an adjunct to conventional treatment. In addition, this form of nutrition therapy reduces the side effects from chemotherapy.

The bottom line is that you should aim for good metabolic health through good nutrition and exercise, which may reduce the risk of developing metabolic dysfunction and cancer.

PREGNANCY'S CONTRIBUTION TO LATER CHRONIC DISEASES

As mentioned previously, certain events during pregnancy (or present in the couple before pregnancy) are known to predispose to later development of chronic diseases in the offspring. For example, gestational diabetes increases the baby's chance of developing diabetes later.

After meticulous investigative research, Professor David Barker noted a relationship between pregnancy and subsequent health problems like heart disease (death from heart attacks) and type 2 diabetes in later adult life. I was a young obstetrician when I saw his influential article in the *British Medical Journal* in 1988. His theory that there were influences during pregnancy that had lifelong impacts on the development of heart and diabetic disease later was the foundation of the 'fetal origins of adult disease' hypothesis discussed in chapter six.

PREVENTION PLAYBOOK
CHAPTER SUMMARY

Maintaining normal insulin levels must be a major goal in your efforts to support your body's requirements and attain or maintain good health.

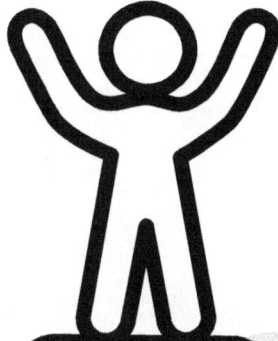

Part 3

REACH THE SUMMIT

(PUT THE PLAYBOOK INTO ACTION)

"In the end, it's not the years in your life that count. It's the life in your years."

– Abraham Lincoln

Chapter 13

SAFEGUARD YOUR
FUTURE HEALTH

**"Good, better, best. Never let it rest.
'Til your good is better and
your better is best."**
– St Jerome

Congratulations, you have started your journey to learn the essentials of caring for your body and health and reduce your risk of developing the unnecessary burden of chronic diseases. By reading this book, you have become aware of the drivers of good health, taking advantage of my years of involvement in health matters. You accept that you must become your own instructor, the student, and the beneficiary. This is your journey, and you report to yourself. You have read and understand what the drivers of both good and poor health are, and you have decided to act. But first – plan.

In motivation and self-help books, they suggest you think about previous efforts to achieve a goal. Maybe it was to lose some weight. Think about what helped you achieve your goal – or, alternatively, what stopped you from achieving your goal.

There are suggestions to use the **SMART** approach when goal setting:

- **S**pecific
- **M**easurable
- **A**chievable
- **R**ealistic
- **T**ime-bound

You can certainly follow such a plan. You may wish to improve your nutrition, lose some weight, or become fitter. Imposing a specific measurement goal like weight loss, or a timeframe for achieving another health goal, is laudable, but what then? Where to first?

If you agree with my idea of supporting your body's requirements, and curtailing the lifestyle risk factors, then *this should become a lifelong mission*, and the results in weight and fitness will follow. You will need to consider whether your plan is achievable and realistic for you. However, you don't need to become a martyr to the cause, as little 'holidays' from your new health approach to life are unlikely to be a catastrophe. Start slowly.

Why should you bother?

Because...

a. It is not difficult!

b. Maintaining good health is an investment in your future.

c. Your good health is a resource to keep you fully functional for as long as possible.

d. You would prefer to retain independence as you age.

e. The health-*care* system is struggling under the weight of so much chronic disease.

f. You were made to believe that the science of nutrition was settled, when in fact there was strong evidence of contradictions in the prevailing dogma, which should have made those recommendations redundant.

g. There is other scientific evidence that leads to the good health outcomes you seek.

* * *

To safeguard your future health, you will need to take four specific actions:

1. Be aware of what your body requires for healthy function

and good health.

2. Be aware of what can damage your health.

3. Determine your present health status.

4. Take control.

ACTION 1 – BE AWARE OF WHAT YOUR BODY REQUIRES FOR HEALTHY FUNCTION AND GOOD HEALTH

What does your body require from you to have all systems and processes working efficiently?

In summary, the four principal factors are:

a. Nourishment. Maintenance of normal metabolism and homeostasis through good nutrition choices.

b. Movement. Maintenance of muscular and joint health to help you mobilise without difficulty.

c. Recovery. Restore mind, memory, and body through adequate sleep, and self-restoration activities to reduce stress.

d. Engagement. Socialisation and engagement with nature. Have purpose in your daily life.

Nourishment

As mentioned at the beginning of the book, in Australia, 26 percent of children and more than 60 percent of adults are overweight or obese.[1] I am not being critical of people in this situation, as knowledge and circumstances may be against them. However, the probability is that metabolic function may be already compromised for many of these individuals.

Most of those adults and children will have Insulin resistance and hyperinsulinaemia. It is likely that their nutrition could be improved. Diets are marketed as solutions… but are you aware that almost any of the common diets will help with weight loss, at least for a while? Making better food choices (this usually means cutting out sugar, refined grains like flour, and ultra-processed foods) is always beneficial. Diets that involve severe calorie restriction are usually not sustainable, resulting in yo-yo dieting, and, for many, it is all too difficult to continue. Fatigue is common. Motivation is often compromised. Negative mood changes are virtually inevitable. Another real problem is the constant feeling of hunger (that is why I call severe calorie restriction a 'starvation' diet). When the weight target is reached and the starvation diet is ceased, often there is a return to bad food choices. Then rapid weight gain is inevitable, and sometimes you can end up heavier than before commencing the diet.

I am very impressed with the studies behind nutrition choices based on an omnivore diet of:

- Low carbohydrates (less that 50 to 100 g per day, mostly above-ground leafy greens, berries, no sugars, no starches, no refined-flour foods like bread, no ultra-processed food)
- Healthy fats (avocados, olives, cream, and cheese)
- Average to high protein (animal-sourced)

These *real food* options are a lifestyle choice that offers adequate variety, are satiating and nourishing, and incorporate all the essential fatty acids, amino acids, and micronutrients. Often, eating episodes per day are less because of satiety and become based on genuine need to eat rather than swings in glucose.

Variations on low-carbohydrate eating include time-restricted eating, ketogenic diet, and intermittent fasting. The carnivore diet – that is, meat only – demands a great commitment. However, I am aware of many people who swear that their brain and physical health improved dramatically on the diet.

I have no axe to grind with nonbelievers in the importance of animal products. But if you plan to avoid animal products entirely, I suggest consulting a dietician who should emphasise the need for a wide variety of plant-based foods to ensure long-term health. Vegetarians and vegans should monitor iron, vitamin B12, and other micronutrients now before potential deficiencies lead to poor health.

Recently, my wife showed me some photos from 14 years ago, taken at a swimming spot while walking in New Zealand. It was almost embarrassing to see my protruding abdomen. I was 14 kg heavier than I am now, even though I thought I was fit. It was just before the penny dropped for both of us that it was time to take a different approach to our nutrition. Breakfast cereals, bread, pasta, pizza, rice, potatoes, and my favourite soft drinks were taken off our 'eat in moderation' dietary approach. Coffee with pouring cream and tea without sugar became bearable after a few days. Blood pressure and weight improved over weeks to months.

Not surprisingly, I now have a bias towards low-carbohydrate nutrition. Average carbohydrate consumption for Australians is about 200 to 300 g per day.[2] Low carbohydrate means eating less than 100 g per day, but preferably less than 50 g. Some people will go to even lower intake, that is, follow a keto diet (and will enter physiological ketosis, a fat-burning state!). When eating low carbohydrate, and especially when fasting or in ketosis, your body burns fats for energy.

I am not militant about my sugar intake. I still have a little birthday cake on each of the grandchildren's special days, and I eat whatever delicious meal is served at dinner parties so I do not put pressure on the hosts. But mostly, I eat real food, above-ground vegetables and leafy greens, fish, meat, eggs, and berries, along with a piece of fruit or some cheese for a snack when needed. I still have a problem with chocolate – I do not buy it, but I devour it if it is offered. I could do better with wine, but often I have two or three alcohol-free nights during the week. I find that two meals per day is usually enough, so, by accident, I have been practising time-restricted eating or inter-mittent fasting.

Movement

I discussed exercise in chapter five. It is as powerful as many med-ications in managing health. But as you may have heard, "You can't outrun a bad diet." For many people, daily life has become less active and more sedentary. Exercise in any form promotes better health for mitochondria, improved energy usage, and mobility maintenance. Exercise is associated with longer health span and aids recovery from physical and mental health issues. If you are not used to exercise, start slowly.

Look up 'zone 2' training. Walking or jogging at a pace that allows easy conversation has a great impact on mitochondria and, therefore, metabolic health. As mentioned previously, repeated 2-minute walks throughout the day may be as beneficial as an all-at-once 60-minute session. Resistance training using bodyweight or weights in a gym adds strength, which promotes new muscle fibre growth and increased numbers of better-functioning mitochondria, along with an improved ability to uptake glucose.

Recovery

Too busy? Overstressed? Are you a worrier who ruminates about what is happening today and might happen tomorrow?

Even if it is for only 15 minutes in a quiet safe room, a walk in nature, watching the clouds, listening to the birds, observing the seasons' changes in the trees and flowers, your mind will become distracted. Your mind and body will relish those moments to self-restore, gather your breath, and prepare you to go back to the grind of daily living. Maybe arrange a massage, an aromatherapy session, learn about controlled breathing and mindfulness. Drop the phone, forget social media, do not look at emails or news bites. Maybe even forget about the distant wars and other atrocities, if only for 15 minutes.

Engagement

Contact a friend or a social or community group. Walking, jogging, book club, bridge club – there are plenty of possibilities. These social interactions create purpose and distraction, as well as brain activity. Take regular trips to parks, into the country-side, along a riverbank, or to the beach. These are re-energising, restorative activities that create stimulation, enjoyment, distrac-tion. Our own thoughts can be introspective. They need to be released to explore some of nature's wonders.

ACTION 2 – BE AWARE OF WHAT CAN DAMAGE YOUR HEALTH

In chapter six, I discussed the drivers of poor health. Some determinants of chronic diseases have genetic or familial predis-positions, while others are dependent on social, economic, and political determinants that are beyond your immediate control. However, there are drivers over which you do have control.

I believe that to successfully achieve your best health, you must consider avoiding lifestyle choices that carry poor health consequences over time.

For example, you already know the impact of excess alcohol, smoking, vaping, and illicit drug use. They will cause negative health consequences in time.

Let's add to the information about alcohol in chapter six.

What should you do? How should you approach alcohol consumption? Let me give you a guide.

Australian recommendations suggest four or fewer standard drinks (40 g alcohol) per day and less than ten standard drinks (100 g) per week.

- 1 standard drink = 10 g of alcohol.
- 375 ml bottle of full-strength beer = 1.4 standard drinks.
- 100 ml glass of wine (red/white/champagne) = 1 standard drink.
- Bottle of wine (red/white/champagne) = 7 to 8 standard drinks.
- 30 ml glass of spirits (40 percent alcohol) = 1 standard drink.

Personally, I love to have one or two glasses of wine most nights. I am retired, do not drive afterwards, and have no responsibility to look after children. I do not consume enough to have terribly interrupted sleep, or a hangover to ruin the next day. My liver enzyme markers for liver inflammation are in the optimum range.

Your decision; your choice. No excess. Keep an eye on metabolic function and dysfunction markers through regular screening.

I cannot recommend other behavioural risks, such as smoking, vaping, or 'recreational' drugs.

It can be very exciting to be spontaneous and do something

on the spur of the moment. You hear about the new weight loss drug, the new health approach your friends are talking about, the great new health guru who has an appealing podcast – and sells a few supplements too. You know the saying, "If it sounds too good to be true…"

ACTION 3 – DETERMINE YOUR PRESENT HEALTH STATUS

Is there evidence of metabolic dysfunction?

Health Spectrum Barometer

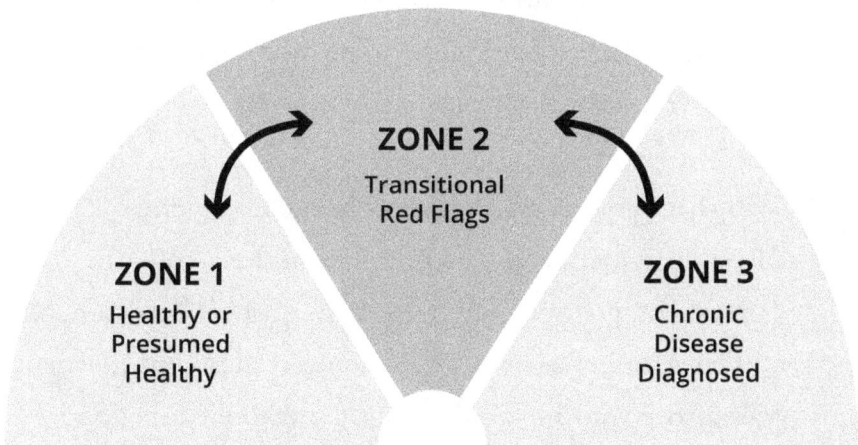

ZONE 2
Transitional
Red Flags

ZONE 1
Healthy or
Presumed
Healthy

ZONE 3
Chronic
Disease
Diagnosed

Each zone can transition, deteriorate, or improve.

You can determine where your health destiny is headed. Is it staying in or returning to better health? Or is it moving towards chronic disease?

Sometimes you just know. You have a feeling that you could be healthier. Of course, if you are aware of any significant family medical problems like heart disease, dementia, cancer, or diabetes, it will pay dividends to discuss these with your doctor. You may have one of the Red Flag conditions I discussed in chapter seven, such as weight gain, gestational diabetes, PCOS, hypertension, erection difficulties, or mental health problems like anxiety. Are you noticing clothes are tighter, especially around the midriff? Two-thirds of Australians, and even more in some other countries, are overweight if not obese, so you are not alone.[3] If you have a Red Flag condition, it suggests your body is already trying to cope with metabolic problems.

There are a few simple measurements that will give you a baseline, and these can be done at home and repeated after any intervention you decide to make.

1. **Weight**. Being overweight may be a consequence of reduced metabolic function. If you think you are overweight, good nutrition, exercise, and good sleep habits will have an impact in time. When you start your journey to improve your metabolic health, metabolic function heals quickly within days to weeks. Weight will take a little longer.

2. **Abdominal circumference**. Australian waist measurement recommendations are < 80 cm for an adult female and < 94 cm for an adult male (the US figures are higher).[4] These are ideal goals. Higher measurements may

reflect abnormal fat accumulation around your abdominal organs (visceral fat), a marker of reduced metabolic function. If your measurements are higher, consider your action plan straight away.

You may also check your waist circumference in relation to your height or hips as mentioned in chapter seven.

3. **Blood pressure (BP).** The commonest reasons for elevated blood pressure are metabolic dysfunction and chronic stress. Consider buying a home blood pressure monitor. They are cheap, can be bought in chemists, and are easy to use.

   Interpretation of what constitutes abnormal blood pressure has changed, with the levels now suggesting aiming for lower than 120/80. You do not have to know what systolic and diastolic measurements mean; the machine will display them. Measurements are best taken after a little rest, in a comfortable chair, with no distraction that might make you tense. Persistent levels above 140/90 should be mentioned to your doctor. Some people with higher levels can be fitted with a 24-hour monitor. BP measurements are taken continuously as you go about your normal daily chores, and during sleep. The average pressure is used to indicate if there is hypertension.

Consult Your Doctor and Get Blood Tests

Even if you feel perfectly well, visiting your doctor − perhaps annually – is a good idea. After discussion and examination, your doctor may recommend a blood test. If not, you can ask for a general blood evaluation for:

a. Routine screening for general health markers
b. Metabolic health screening

A 'routine' blood test usually includes blood count profile – for example, testing for anaemia – and ESR (erythrocyte sedimentation rate) or CRP (C-reactive protein) – for example, checking for evidence of inflammation. Kidney and liver function as well as biochemical measurements like sodium, glucose, and cholesterol will give you and your doctor a reasonable overview of your health state. Vitamin D should also be assessed, as it has many essential functions in the body. Unfortunately, many Australians have suboptimal levels. If any of these results are abnormal, your doctor will explain and advise on management.

I firmly believe that metabolic health screening should be carried out from your 20s or 30s and thereafter. Presently, this is not part of a nationally recommended screening program.

If metabolic dysfunction is the major contributor or indeed causative pathology for most of the chronic diseases, suboptimal test results may lead to taking action many years, even decades, before dysfunction overwhelms the body's ability to adapt, and a chronic disease is diagnosed.

Prevention may save you from a subsequent diagnosis and future consequences.

Extra tests I suggest are:

- Fasting glucose
- Fasting insulin
- HbA1c
- Liver enzymes GGT, AST, ALT

When the results are available, check your scores against the pathology laboratory's range. I have a principle that if a test lies just within the 'normal' range, it may not be optimum. Middle range is better than high normal values. Ask for a copy of your results so you can make comparisons with future tests.

Additional Health Status Assessments to Consider

When identifying your present health status, there are a couple of additional assessments that can help paint a clearer picture.

Consider trialling a CGM (Continuous Glucose Monitor)

Have you heard about CGM? The CGM device is recommended for individuals with type 1 diabetes. Some also recommend its use for individuals living with type 2 diabetes. Personally, I believe CGM to be useful for anyone who is keen to learn their body's response to their food choices. It is a small device that is painless to apply to your arm or abdomen. It registers your blood glucose levels continuously and can relay this information to your mobile phone. It may replace the need for fingerprick blood glucose assessments.

You may be one of the few people who do not get glucose spikes from breakfast cereals, rice, pasta, bananas, and bread. But if you are like most people, your glucose will probably spike to a high level after some meals. For example, a bowl of oats with some berries for breakfast is often recommended because it can lower LDL cholesterol. However, you may be surprised at the glucose spike. Noting the effect of different fruits can be quite instructive. Berries are the safest, and one banana is equivalent to ingesting several spoonfuls of sugar. The glucose spike after starchy foods (normal or sweet potatoes, rice, pasta) will be much higher compared to green leafy salad vegetables. And of course, watch the response to burgers, soft drinks, fruit juices, takeaway meals, alcohol, and exercise.

Every glucose spike in your body is followed quickly by a rise in insulin. If you have breakfast, morning tea/coffee with a biscuit or banana bread, lunch, afternoon tea (with a small biscuit), evening meal, and occasionally a snack before bedtime, glucose levels will spike frequently, but insulin levels will probably remain elevated. That is hyperinsulinaemia, and you have learnt that persistently raised serum insulin has detrimental effects on every blood vessel in the body. Your metabolism will eventually struggle, and you will increase the risk of developing one of the chronic diseases.

Consider measuring your CACS (coronary artery calcium score)

Nearly all of my 50- to 70-year-old friends have had this test carried out. Indeed, the presence of calcium in the coronary arteries can be noticed in some 20-year-olds, but is present in 90 percent of men (less in women) over age 70.[5] The test is not supported by Medicare. Indeed, many doctors, including cardiologists, argue against having it carried out for several reasons, including cost, radiation exposure, and the potential for inaccuracies.

The test is a form of special X-ray that is sometimes combined with a specialised CT scan of the heart blood vessels. If the test shows no calcium in your heart arteries, it means that there is no arterial disease present, and the potential to have a heart attack during the following 10 years is minimal. A score from 1 to 99 suggests mild heart artery disease, 100 to 399 suggests moderate, and above 400 reflects severe coronary artery disease and high risk for heart attack or another major adverse cardiac event sometime in the future.

Calcium settles in areas of damage or inflammation, and after its deposition assists with the subsequent repair in the artery. It accumulates in plaques, which can get bigger with repeated damage and eventually reduce or stop blood flow through the artery.

The presence of calcium in the heart arteries is a reflection of past accumulation of calcium for whatever reason, and while it probably cannot be reversed, it is possible to stop the score rising further. This can be achieved by actively using the drivers of good health (nourishment – especially low-carbohydrate eating – movement, recovery, engagement) and actively stopping the drivers that degrade your health (for example, smoking, alcohol excess, substance abuse, weight gain).

If your CACS is high, your doctor may discuss your blood pressure, run blood tests for metabolic dysfunctions like diabetes and high cholesterol, and refer you to a cardiologist.

ACTION 4 – TAKE CONTROL

**You are the best person to plan
for your future health.**

Your body is complex. Expecting that health can be ignored for the moment and only become an issue when mortality is questioned is all too common. It is a mistake, I believe, to avoid taking steps to look after your body, expecting that the development of any chronic disease will be remedied by Australia's lauded healthcare system. By the time you need the doctors and nurses and other healthcare practitioners, most of the chronic diseases will have already overcome your amazingly adaptable body systems. Medications or surgery may alleviate symptoms and signs and keep up the appearance of health – but who wants diabetes, dementia, or cancer that could have been prevented? Wear and tear will come with aging, but to recall Professor David Barker's quote, "Chronic diseases are unnecessary."

As mentioned previously, the confusion and conflict in the health arena includes corporate and political agendas. I am not naive to the social and economic dilemmas that are being faced by so many Australians, and these are mostly outside their control. I know they add to mental and physical health impacts. I know how difficult it is for new parents, mothers especially. I know that work and travel times make some people time-poor.

Doctors are aware that lifestyle habits can sabotage health. However, through experience, they also know that people often request 'quick fixes' and lack the motivation to change long-entrenched lifestyle habits. There is no doubt that prescribed medicines have a role in managing chronic diseases and acute health conditions. However, for some people, there will be side effects that can have negative impacts that outweigh the expected benefits. Correct use of prescribed medications is mandatory, and suspected side effects should be reported immediately. Some people are prescribed several drugs to be taken 1 to 3 or 4 times per day. For older people in particular, confusion can lead to failure to take the tablets, or doubling up. Problems from medications are a common cause of hospital admissions.

My personal opinion is that medications are prescribed (and sought) too quickly. It is not an insult to your doctor if you ask for more details about your need for medication and the expected benefits and side effects. There are so many instances of medications being withdrawn (sometimes years after their release into the market) because of 'unexpected' dangers. New medications come to the market and are 'tried' on people willing to get a pill cure for their complaint. The 'next big thing' isn't always as good or as safe as its marketing would suggest.

In as much as you have control and are willing to take stock of your present health state, and if you are willing to make your health a real goal, you, perhaps with the help of your doctor, can trial behaviour changes instead of starting a medication, and monitor the outcome. Which changes? I repeat – better nutrition, more movement (exercise), better sleep hygiene and self-restoration practices, more social engagement, minimising alcohol, avoiding smoking, vaping, and illicit drugs.

TAKE CONTROL

- ✅ Better nutrition

- ✅ More movement

- ✅ Better sleep hygiene

- ✅ More self-restoration practices

- ✅ Minimise alcohol

- ✅ Avoid smoking-vaping-illicit drugs

- ✅ Assess metabolic health now and occasionally (maybe 2-5 yearly)

- ✅ Do not ignore 'Red Flags'

George Bernard Shaw said, "Life wasn't meant to be easy, my child; but take courage: it can be delightful." May I add, life will be easier if you give time to maintain or achieve health.

PREVENTION PLAYBOOK
CHAPTER SUMMARY

———————

My strong conviction is that preventative healthcare should include early screening for metabolic function and dysfunction.

In as much as you have control and are willing to take stock of your present health state, and if you are willing to make your health a real goal, you, perhaps with the help of your doctor, can trial behaviour changes instead of starting a medication, and monitor the outcome.

"Twenty years from now you will be more disappointed by the things you didn't do than by the ones you did do."

– H Jackson Brown Jr

Chapter 14

FINAL THOUGHTS

The human life cycle commences as one tiny cell in the womb. Death is the inevitable end. We should not fear it. It just does not seem right, however, if deteriorating health from chronic diseases means 10 to 20 years of poor-quality daily living, taking an array of medications daily, and still dying a decade younger than expected from the life cycle. This is what is happening to too many Australians. The information is available on how to optimise your health and reduce or possibly eliminate the risk of chronic disease.

Where are you in your journey? You may have aging parents who are becoming dependent on your help, or a friend diagnosed with cancer or memory lapses. And if you have a young family, work commitments, and are suffering from sleep deprivation, there is little time to concentrate on your own wellbeing. It becomes difficult to manage healthy eating and exercise. You visit your doctor because of stress, anxiety, insomnia, 'burnout', and you are prescribed some medication. Yes, now you think it is time to start taking better care of yourself and concentrating on your own health. But where to start?

Making Sense of Health was written in the aftermath of realising I needed to think about my own mortality. The chest pain was not severe, just persistent. All bloods, the chest X-ray, and ECG were normal. But antacid and analgesics did not work. My friend, a cardiologist, suggested an angiogram to check my coronary arteries. Lo and behold, to our surprise, one main artery (often nicknamed the 'widow maker') was virtually completely blocked. He inserted a stent, and the next morning I declared that I would now be unstoppable at running club and gym!

But honestly, full recovery and confidence took some months. Now I can say that my energy is back to normal. I so enjoyed playing soccer with our 4-year-old grandson, riding the Alps 2 Ocean bicycle track on New Zealand's South Island with several friends, and regularly pushing myself at the gym or jogging. Without any doubt, some advances in the surgical world have been outstanding, and I for one am truly grateful. Thank you, Guy!

Reflecting on reasons why I had a heart artery blockage, I realise there were several contributing factors. I now realise that I had metabolic dysfunction, and likely the frequently associated problems of systemic chronic inflammation and chronic stress. I ignored the Red Flags, the warning signs of abdominal weight gain, poor sleep patterns, job 'demands', years of passive smoking. I do think that if, 20 or 30 years ago, I had known what I know now, what I have written about in this book, it is probable that things would have been different.

What about you? Has this book stirred a desire to put into practice good nutrition, plenty of exercise, healthy sleep hygiene, and, importantly, give yourself time for mind restoration? I hope you now know what the body wants from you, as well as what your body would prefer not to be forced to cope with. It is up to you. Yes, doctors and other healthcare practitioners can help. Government strategies to improve the nation's health can also help – if they are put into action. But your personal efforts are needed to prevent disease development, especially to control metabolic health. Become proactive. Take control of your health destiny. The dividends will be worth it.

I hope this book is just what you needed. I hope you can make better sense of the challenging subject of health. Less confusion. No didactic lectures about what you have neglected, the time lost, and what you *must* do from now. Instead, you now have information to give you awareness around health. Continue to build your knowledge so you can determine what will work for you.

PREVENTION PLAYBOOK
CHAPTER SUMMARY

Metabolic dysfunction is a major root cause
or contributing pathology of cardiovascular
disease, cerebral vascular disease, dementia,
hypertension, nephropathy, retinopathy, penile
erectile dysfunction, peripheral vascular
disease, gestational diabetes, peripheral
and central neuropathy, and more.

Epilogue

———————

TIME IN NATURE

While writing a section of this book, I was sitting outside on a beautiful warm, sunny day, under the shade of a jacaranda tree in full bloom and listening to some small Australian bird singing away in a nearby bush. Yes, I am privileged, and this is quite a luxury. Retirement has its perks.

Being in nature is so stimulating yet calming, a distraction. I re-read Wordsworth's poem, 'I Wandered Lonely as a Cloud' and felt his joy as he proclaimed, "And then my heart with pleasure fills. And dances with the daffodils." I think of plants and animals, no matter how big or small, and the fact that they all started out as one tiny cell with a nucleus containing their DNA and those special entities called mitochondria. As each cell grows, divides, and differentiates, the final plant or animal in its mature form will contribute to the 10 million different species of living organisms that populate the oceans and streams and land masses of Mother Earth. Those magnificent nature documentaries never fail to engender excitement at the diversity in nature, of which humans are a small part.

Locally, there may be nothing more exciting than a barking dog, birds quarrelling in the sky, or a beautiful butterfly zigzagging through the garden. Oh yes, and the occasional pesky mosquito or fly. How is it that when you start slicing a roast chicken in the kitchen, one or more of these creatures come at great speed to annoy you as they explore their chances of sustenance?

Underground in the soil, there is another world of life that we often do not think about. The roots of all plants, trees, and flowers venture from the main trunks in search of minerals and water to add to the energy they receive from the sun and our exhaled carbon dioxide. In the soil, the roots encounter and communicate with organisms that provide necessary nutrients and aid growth. There are hyphae of fungi spreading through the soil, working in symbiosis with each other and with plants. In one cubic metre of fertile soil, there are a billion other living creatures. Some you can see, like earthworms, termites, and millipedes, but most you cannot see, for example, bacteria, actinomyces, and algae. And each one, no matter how tiny, has its own life cycle and purpose. They may be aerators of the soil, nutrient providers to plants, or decomposers of leaf litter, wood, dead animals, and animal excrement. Their existence contributes to the magnificent ecosystem of planet Earth.

When plants are healthy, with adequate sunlight, soil, water, and nutrients, they usually thrive. Given poor soil, excessively dry weather, or when attacked by pests, they become unhealthy. When eventually they die, they in turn are decomposed and become contributors to the energy and nutrient cycles.

We humans are so similar to all other organisms. Sir David Attenborough reminds us that, "We share the Earth with the living world – the most remarkable life-support system imaginable."

**Nature is there to excite and delight,
to distract when necessary.**

With good nourishment, humans will usually thrive, even though we are at the mercy of our genetics and need plenty of sleep and movement, along with that special need to have socialisation and purpose.

We are vulnerable, however, to temporary deteriorations in health from infections or injury. The body's resources include a magnificent surveillance system to identify the attacking organism or injury and set about repairing the problem. Additionally, events in life may make us sad, anxious, or emotional. But again, these should be considered part and parcel of normal life, and, more often than not, we cope and adapt. However, there are factors that can exert a strain on the body's resources, which can overwhelm its ability to cope, reducing our health state to poor health and leading to many consequences. These are the drivers of disease. You have met them in the pages of this book, and now you understand them.

Your job, should you choose to take it, is to do all you can to support the special requirements of your treasured body.

PREVENTION PLAYBOOK
ROUND-UP

Health is a concept – difficult to define, something we want, especially when we lose it, desirable yet variable, an expectation yet not guaranteed, a matter of strongly held opinions and confusion.

It is not unreasonable to expect long-term health. By using the drivers of good health, by giving your body the essential support it needs from nourishment, movement, recovery, and engagement socially and with nature, you will maintain or return to better health.

Long-term chronic diseases are all too common. Modern medicine may assist by providing newer medications, but

I believe the expectation of lifelong
health must be accompanied by taking
personal responsibility, that is, making
a commitment to prevention.

Reliable information is knowledge. Health
knowledge gives you the opportunity
to safeguard your health destiny.

―――――――――

There is abundant but conflicting health
information. In our compromised and
conflicted world, not only is it difficult
to make sense of it all, but you must
become aware of the many influences
and biases in health advice or risk
becoming an easy target for those who
wish to capitalise on our naivety.

―――――――――

In the normal healthy physiological
state, the processes of metabolism,

immune reaction, and stress
responses work together to maintain
homeostasis and normal health.

———————

Dysfunction of bodily processes,
particularly metabolic dysfunction,
contributes to all of the chronic
diseases – cardiovascular disease,
cerebral vascular disease, dementia,
hypertension, nephropathy, retinopathy,
peripheral vascular disease, gestational
diabetes, type 2 diabetes, peripheral
and central neuropathy, and more.

———————

Maintaining or restoring normal
metabolic function must be the
priority of healthcare and healing.

———————

There are several recognisable Red
Flags that are indicative of metabolic

dysfunction and therefore predict
future poor health. If uncorrected, the
inevitable outcome is a chronic disease.

———————

Normal insulin production is
necessary for healthy metabolism
and good health.

———————

The core pathology of metabolic
dysfunction is resistance to the
actions of insulin (insulin resistance).
This creates excessive insulin production
(hyperinsulinaemia), which has
detrimental effects on every blood
vessel in the body, as well as
promoting type 2 diabetes and
other chronic diseases.

———————

Maintaining normal insulin levels
must be a major goal in your efforts

to support your body's requirements
and attain or maintain good health.

———————

Food choices have a direct impact
on insulin levels and metabolism.

———————

Type 2 diabetes can be reversed
and prevented with dietary changes,
especially by reducing carbohydrate-
heavy foods, particularly restricting
foods that contain simple carbohydrates
(bread, pasta, rice), avoiding regular
fruit juice drinks, ultra-processed foods
(UPFs), foods with added sugar, and
foods cooked using seed oils (used in
UPFs, fast food, and home cooking).

———————

Because the pathology of most chronic
diseases has the same contributing
pathways as type 2 diabetes, there

is hope that a similar dietary
approach will aid in the prevention
or remission of these diseases.

———————

Preventative healthcare should
include early screening for metabolic
function and dysfunction. For people
who have warning signs of metabolic
dysfunction (Red Flags), or any of the
chronic diseases, severe carbohydrate
restriction should be their goal.

———————

You are the best person to take control of
the factors that promote good health.

ACKNOWLEDGEMENTS

I am so grateful to all at Dean Publishing but particularly my editor Matt Moore, my cover and format designer Jazmine Morales, and Natalie Deane who offered great encouragement after accepting the first draft.

Thank you to Alan Kennedy, Carol Newton, and Dr Stephen Shepherd, who read a very early draft – their advice helped me enormously. And then there is Sue Tonakie, who knows as much about nutrition and medications as leaders in those disciplines. Sue was a hugely important silent editor of my first book *Our Children, Our Legacy*. Together, we continue to try and make sense of health.

Finally, I am part of a running group. These friends have put up with my monologues every session (hoping I'd run out of breath!). Thank you Therese, Adam, Bill, Brett, Jaimie, Steve.

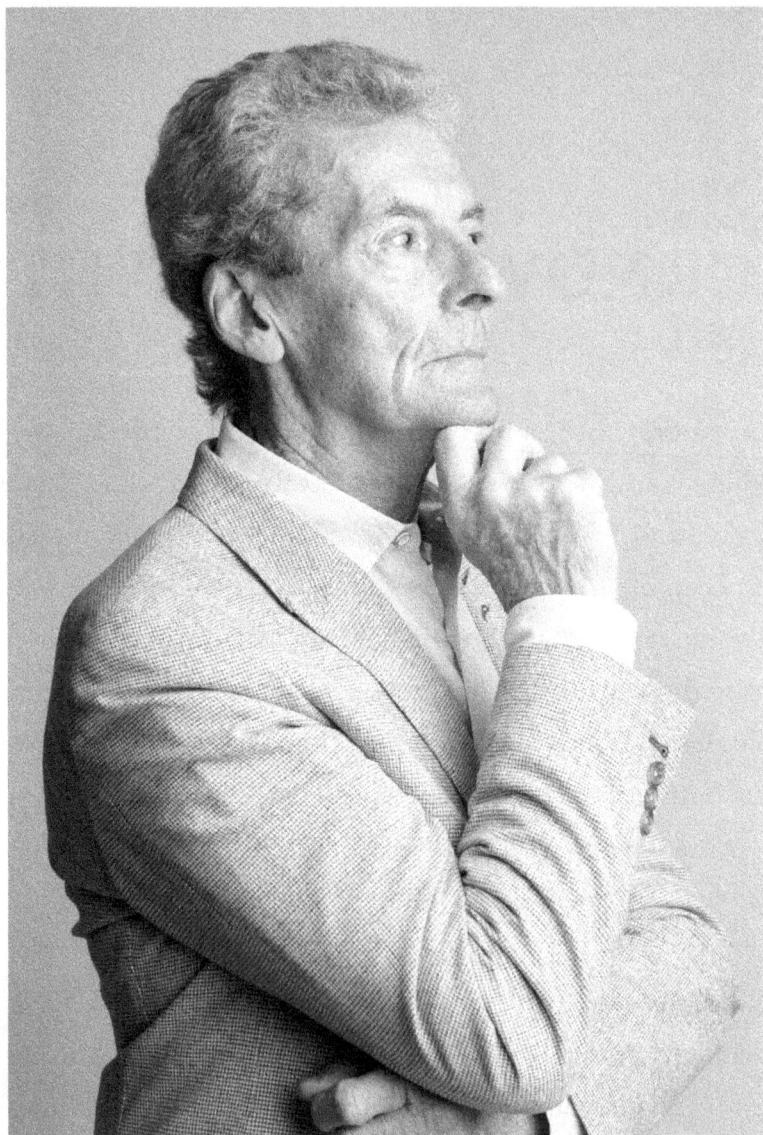

ABOUT THE AUTHOR

Dr Tim O'Dowd is an author, researcher, and retired obstetrician, gynaecologist, and fertility and IVF specialist, as well as a husband, father, and grandfather. He also holds a Master of Palliative Care. In 2021, he published his first book, *Our Children, Our Legacy: Passing on the Gift of Good Health.*

After a medical scare prompted him to re-examine his own health, Tim's research led him to discover that much of what he thought he knew about maintaining and safeguarding health was wrong. With the science of health constantly changing, his latest mission is to help people understand the drivers of chronic disease and the pillars of good health from an evidence-based perspective. He believes that the best person to safeguard your future health is you.

ENDNOTES

Preface

1 Australian Bureau of Statistics 2023, 'Health Conditions Prevalence', viewed 3 December 2024, https://www.abs.gov.au/statistics/health/health-conditions-and-risks/health-conditions-prevalence/latest-release.

2 Barker, DJP 2012, 'Developmental Origins of Chronic Disease', *Public Health*, vol 126, no 3, pp 185–189, doi.org/10.1016/j.puhe.2011.11.014.

3 Smith, R 2003, 'Thoughts for New Medical Students at a New Medical School', *British Medical Journal*, 327, pp 1430–1433, doi.org/10.1136/bmj.327.7429.1430.

4 Hallberg, SJ, Gershuni, VM, Hazbun, TL, & Athinarayanan, SJ 2019, 'Reversing Type 2 Diabetes: A Narrative Review of the Evidence', *Nutrients*, vol 11, no 4, p 766, doi.org/10.3390/nu11040766.

Chapter 1

1 Australian Bureau of Statistics 2024, 'Life Expectancy', viewed 3 December 2024, https://www.abs.gov.au/statistics/people/population/life-expectancy/latest-release.

2 World Health Organization n.d., 'Constitution', viewed 9 December 2024, https://www.who.int/about/governance/constitution.

3 Sartorius, N 2006, 'The Meanings of Health and its Promotion', *Croatian Medical Journal*, vol 47, no 4, pp 662–664. https://pmc.ncbi.nlm.nih.gov/articles/PMC2080455/.

Chapter 2

1 Australian Bureau of Statistics 2023, 'National Health Survey', viewed 12 December 2024, https://www.abs.gov.au/statistics/health/health-conditions-and-risks/national-health-survey/2022; Australian Institute of Health and Welfare 2024, 'Chronic Conditions', *Australian Government*, viewed 12 December 2024, https://www.aihw.gov.au/reports/australias-health/chronic-conditions.

2 Australian Institute of Health and Welfare 2024, 'Older Australians', *Australian Government*, viewed 12 December 2024, https://www.aihw.gov.au/reports/older-people/older-australians/contents/health/

health-disability-status.

3   Department of Health 2021, 'National Preventive Health Strategy',
     Australian Government, viewed 12 December 2024, https://www.health.gov.
     au/resources/publications/national-preventive-health-strategy-2021-2030.

Chapter 3

1   Fischetti, M and Christiansen, J 2021, 'Our Bodies Replace
     Billions of Cells Every Day', *Scientific America,* viewed 19
     December 2024, https://www.scientificamerican.com/article/
     our-bodies-replace-billions-of-cells-every-day/.

2   Chew, NWS, Ng, CH, Tan, DJH, et al. 2019, 'The Global Burden of
     Metabolic Disease: Data from 2000 to 2019', *Cell Metabolism,* vol 3, pp
     414-428, doi.org/10.1016/j.cmet.2023.02.003

Chapter 5

1   Bailey, RL, Leidy, HJ, Mattes, RD, Heymsfield, SB, Boushey, CJ,
     Ahluwalia, N, Cowan, AE, Pannucci, TR, Moshfegh, AJ, Goldman, JD,
     Rhodes, DG, Stoody, EE, de Jesus, J, and Casavale, KO 2022, 'Frequency
     of Eating in the US Population: A Narrative Review of the 2020 Dietary
     Guidelines Advisory Committee Report,' *Current Developments in Nutrition,*
     vol 6, no 1, doi.org/10.1093/cdn/nzac132.

2   The University of North Carolina 2018, 'Only 12 Percent of American
     Adults Are Metabolically Healthy, Carolina Study Finds', viewed 13
     January 2025, https://www.unc.edu/posts/2018/11/28/only-12-per-
     cent-of-american-adults-are-metabolically-healthy-carolina-study-finds/.

3   Lloyd, A 2021, 'Financial Treadmill: Aussies Wasting $2.4 Billion on
     Unused Gym Memberships', *Finder,* viewed 13 January 2025, https://www.
     finder.com.au/news/unused-gym-memberships.

4   Munson, M 2024, 'Can You Actually Turn Back the Aging Clock?', *Men's
     Health,* viewed 13 January 2025, https://www.menshealth.com/health/
     a46716994/anti-aging-strategies-worth-it/.

5   Distefano, G and Goodpaster, BH 2018, 'Effects of Exercise and Aging on
     Skeletal Muscle', *Cold Spring Harbor Perspectives in Medicine,* vol 8, no 3, doi.
     org/10.1101/cshperspect.a029785.

6   Ahlskog, JE, Geda, YE, Graff-Radford, NR, and Petersen, RC 2011,
     'Physical Exercise as a Preventive or Disease-Modifying Treatment of
     Dementia and Brain Aging', *Mayo Clinic Proceedings,* vol 86, no 9, pp

876–884, doi.org/10.4065/mcp.2011.0252.

7   Reimers, CD, Knapp, G, and Reimers, AK 2012, 'Does Physical Activity Increase Life Expectancy? A Review of the Literature', *Journal of Aging Research*, doi.org/10.1155/2012/243958.

8   Colberg, SR, Sigal, RJ, Yardley, JE, Riddell, MC, Dunstan, DW, Dempsey, PC, Horton, ES, Castorino, K, and Tate, DF 2016, 'Physical Activity/ Exercise and Diabetes: A Position Statement of the American Diabetes Association,' *Diabetes Care*, vol 39, no 11, pp 2065–2079, doi.org/10.2337/ dc16-1728.

9   Australian Institute of Health and Welfare 2021, 'Sleep Problems as a Risk Factor for Chronic Conditions', *Australian Government*, viewed 13 January 2025, https://www.aihw.gov.au/reports/risk-factors/ sleep-problems-as-a-risk-factor/summary.

10   Walker, M 2017, *Why We Sleep: The New Science of Sleep and Dreams*, Penguin.

11   Delaney, SK, Allison, S, Looi, JC, Bidargaddi, N, and Bastiampillai, T 2019, 'Rapid National Increases in the Hospitalisation of Australian Youth Due to Intentional Self-Harm Between 2008 and 2019', *Australas Psychiatry*, vol 30, no 2, pp 166–170. doi.org/10.1177/10398562211047919.

Chapter 6

1   Australian Bureau of Statistics n.d., 'Prevalence of Chronic Conditions', viewed 16 December 2024, https://www.abs.gov.au/statistics/meas- uring-what-matters/measuring-what-matters-themes-and-indicators/ healthy/prevalence-chronic-conditions.

2   Australian Institute of Health and Welfare 2024, 'Prevalence and Impact of Mental Illness', *Australian Government*, viewed 16 December 2024, https://www.aihw.gov.au/mental-health/overview/ prevalence-and-impact-of-mental-illness.

3   Steel, A, McIntyre, E, Harnett, J, Foley, H, Adams, J, Sibbritt, D, Wardle, J, and Frawley, J 2018, 'Complementary Medicine Use in the Australian Population: Results of a Nationally-Representative Cross-Sectional Survey', *Scientific Reports*, vol 8, doi.org/10.1038/s41598-018-35508-y.

4   Grima, M and Dixon, JB 2013, 'Obesity Recommendations for Management in General Practice and Beyond', *Australian Family Physician*, vol 42, no 8, https://www.racgp.org.au/afp/2013/august/obesity.

5   Department of Health and Aged Care 2021, 'Body Mass Index (BMI) and Waist Measurement', *Australian Government*, viewed 17 December 2024,

https://www.health.gov.au/topics/overweight-and-obesity/bmi-and-waist.

6   Australian Institute of Health and Welfare 2024, 'Overweight and
     Obesity', *Australian Government*, viewed 17 December 2024, https://
     www.aihw.gov.au/reports/overweight-obesity/overweight-and-obesity/
     contents/summary.

7   Warin, M 2019, 'The Politics of Disease: Obesity in Historical
     Perspective', *Australian Journal of General Practice*, vol 48, no 10, https://
     www1.racgp.org.au/ajgp/2019/october/the-politics-of-disease.

8   Australian Institute of Health and Welfare 2024, 'Overweight and
     Obesity', *Australian Government*, viewed 17 December 2024, https://
     www.aihw.gov.au/reports/overweight-obesity/overweight-and-obesity/
     contents/summary.

9   Solan, M 2023, 'Understanding New Weight-Loss Drugs', *Harvard Health
     Publishing*, viewed 17 December 2024, https://www.health.harvard.edu/
     staying-healthy/understanding-new-weight-loss-drugs.

10   American Heart Association News 2016, 'Kids and Added Sugars: How
     Much Is too Much?', *American Heart Association*, viewed 17 December 2024,
     https://www.heart.org/en/news/2023/05/23/kids-and-added-sugars-
     how-much-is-too-much; World Health Organization 2015, 'Guideline:
     Sugars Intake for Adults and Children', viewed 17 December 2024,
     https://iris.who.int/bitstream/handle/10665/149782/97892415490
     28_eng.pdf.

11   Better Health Channel n.d., 'Genes and Genetics Explained', *State
     Government Victoria*, viewed 17 December 2024, https://www.betterhealth.
     vic.gov.au/health/conditionsandtreatments/genes-and-genetics.

12   Garthwaite, C 2008, 'The Effect of In-Utero Conditions on Long Term
     Health: Evidence from the 1918 Spanish Flu Pandemic', *Kellogg School of
     Management*, viewed 17 December 2024, https://www.kellogg.northwest-
     ern.edu/faculty/garthwaite/htm/fetal_stress_garthwaite_053008.pdf;
     Brown, AS, Begg, MD, Gravenstein, S, Shaefer, CA, Wyatt, RJ, Bresnahan,
     M, Babulas, VP, and Susser, ES 2004, 'Serologic Evidence of Prenatal
     Influenza in the Etiology of Schizophrenia', *Archives of General Psychiatry*, vol
     61, no 8, pp 774–780, doi.org/10.1001/archpsyc.61.8.774.

13   Bleker, LS, de Rooij, SR, Painter, RC, Ravelli, AC, and Roseboom,
     TJ 2021, 'Cohort Profile: The Dutch Famine Birth Cohort (DFBC)- A
     Prospective Birth Cohort Study in the Netherlands', *BMJ Open*, vol 11,
     no 3, doi.org/10.1136/bmjopen-2020-042078; Ramirez, D and Haas,
     SA 2022, 'Windows of Vulnerability: Consequences of Exposure Timing
     during the Dutch Hunger Winter', *Population and Development Review*, vol 48,

no 4, pp 959–989, doi.org/10.1111/padr.12513.

14 Lumey, LH 1992, 'Decreased Birthweights in Infants After Maternal in Utero Exposure to the Dutch Famine of 1944–1945', *Paediatric and Perinatal Epidemiology*, vol 6, no 2, pp 240–253, doi.org/10.1111/j.1365-3016.1992. tb00764.x.

15 Australian Institute of Health and Welfare 2023, 'Sports Injury Hospitalisations Return to Pre-COVID Trends', *Australian Government*, viewed 17 December 2024, https:// www.aihw.gov.au/news-media/media-releases/2023/june/ sports-injury-hospitalisations-return-to-pre-covid.

16 World Health Organization 2022, 'No Level of Alcohol Consumption Is Safe for Our Health', viewed 17 December 2024, https://www.who.int/ europe/news-room/04-01-2023-no-level-of-alcohol-consumption-is-safe-for-our-health.

17 Pelucchi, C, Gallus, S, Garavello, W, Bosetti, C, and La Vecchia, C 2006, 'Cancer Risk Associated with Alcohol and Tobacco Use: Focus on Upper Aero-Digestive Tract and Liver', *Alcohol Research & Health*, vol 29, no 3, pp 193–198, https://pmc.ncbi.nlm.nih.gov/articles/PMC6527045/.

18 Walser, T, Cui, X, Yanagawa, J, Lee, JM, Heinrich, E, Lee, G, Sharma, S, and Dubinett, SM 2008, 'Smoking and Lung Cancer: The Role of Inflammation', *Proceedings of the American Thoracic Society*, vol 5, no 8, pp 811–815, doi.org/10.1513/pats.200809-100TH.

19 AHPRA and National Boards 2021, 'Registered Health Practitioners and Students: What You Need to Know About the COVID-19 Vaccine Rollout', viewed 17 December 2024, https://www.ahpra.gov.au/ News/2021-03-09-vaccination-statement.aspx.

20 Australian Institute of Health and Welfare 2024, 'Health Expenditure', *Australian Government*, viewed 17 December 2024, https://www.aihw.gov. au/reports/health-welfare-expenditure/health-expenditure.

21 World Health Organization 2023, 'Noncommunicable Diseases', viewed 18 December 2024, https://www.who.int/news-room/fact-sheets/detail/ noncommunicable-diseases.

22 Office of National Statistics 2022, 'Health State Life Expectancies by National Deprivation Deciles, England: 2018 to 2020', viewed 18 December 2024, https://www.ons.gov.uk/peoplepopulation-andcommunity/healthandsocialcare/healthinequalities/bulletins/ healthstatelifeexpectanciesbyindexofmultipledeprivationimd/2018to2020.

23 National Center for Health Statistics 2024, 'Life Expectancy', viewed 18

December 2024, https://www.cdc.gov/nchs/fastats/life-expectancy.htm; The University of North Carolina 2018, 'Only 12 Percent of American Adults Are Metabolically Healthy, Carolina Study Finds', viewed 18 December 2024, https://www.unc.edu/posts/2018/11/28/only-12-percent-of-american-adults-are-metabolically-healthy-carolina-study-finds/.

24   Hare, MJL, Zhao, Y, Guthridge, S, Burgess, P, Barr, ELM, Ellis, E, Butler, D, Rosser, A, Falhammer, H, and Maple-Brown, LJ 2022, 'Prevalence and Incidence of Diabetes Among Aboriginal People in Remote Communities of the Northern Territory, Australia: A Retrospective, Longitudinal Data-Linkage Study', *BMJ Open*, doi.org/10.1136/bmjopen-2021-059716.

25   Hare, MJL, Barzi, F, Boyle, JA, Guthridge, S, Dyck, RF, Barr, ELM, Singh, G, Falhammar, H, Webster, V, Shaw, JE, and Maple-Brown, LJ 2020, 'Diabetes During Pregnancy and Birthweight Trends Among Aboriginal and Non-Aboriginal People in the Northern Territory of Australia Over 30 Years', *The Lancet Regional Health – Western Pacific*, vol 1, doi.org/10.1016/j.lanwpc.2020.100005.

26   Australian Bureau of Statistics 2024, 'Overseas Migration', viewed 18 December 2024, https://www.abs.gov.au/statistics/people/population/overseas-migration/latest-release.

27   Australian Institute of Health and Welfare 2024, 'Alcohol, Tobacco & Other Drugs in Australia', *Australian Government*, viewed 18 December 2024, https://www.aihw.gov.au/reports/alcohol/alcohol-tobacco-other-drugs-australia/contents/drug-types/tobacco.

28   Standing Committee on Health, Aged Care and Sport 2024, 'The State of Diabetes Mellitus in Australia in 2024', *Parliament of Australia*, viewed 18 December 2024, https://www.aph.gov.au/Parliamentary_Business/Committees/House/Health_Aged_Care_and_Sport/Inquiry_into_Diabetes/Report.

29   Department of Health 2021, 'National Preventive Health Strategy', *Australian Government*, viewed 18 December 2024, https://www.health.gov.au/resources/publications/national-preventive-health-strategy-2021-2030.

30   Department of Health and Aged Care 2021, 'The National Preventive Health Strategy 2021–2030 – What Does it Mean for Australians?', *Australian Government*, viewed 18 December 2024, https://www.health.gov.au/sites/default/files/documents/2021/12/national-preventive-health-strategy-2021-2030-national-preventive-health-strategy-2021-2030-summary.pdf.

31   Department of Health and Aged Care 2022, 'National Obesity Strategy 2022–2032', *Australian Government*, viewed 18 December

2024, https://www.health.gov.au/resources/publications/national-obesity-strategy-2022-2032.

32 Australian Institute of Health and Welfare 2024, 'Overweight and Obesity', *Australian Government*, viewed 18 December 2024, https://www.aihw.gov.au/reports/overweight-obesity/overweight-and-obesity/contents/summary.

33 de Lacy-Vawdon, C, Vandenberg, B, and Livingstone, CH 2022, 'Recognising the Elephant in the Room: The Commercial Determinants of Health', *BMJ Global Health*, vol 7, doi.org/10.1136/bmjgh-2021-007156.

34 Lane, MM, Gamage, E, Du, S, Ashtree, DN, McGuinness, AJ, Gauci, S, Baker, P, Lawrence, M, Rebholz, CM, Srour, B, Touvier, M, Jacka, FN, O'Neill, A, Segasby, T, and Marx, W 2024, 'Ultra-Processed Food Exposure and Adverse Health Outcomes: Umbrella Review of Epidemiological Meta-Analyses', *BMJ*, doi.org/10.1136/bmj-2023-077310.

35 Gornall, J 2015, 'Sugar: Spinning a Web of Influence', *BMJ*, vol 350, doi.org/10.1136/bmj.h231.

36 Aaron, DG and Siegel, MB 2017, 'Sponsorship of National Health Organizations by Two Major Soda Companies', *American Journal of Preventative Medicine*, vol 52, no 1, pp 20–30, doi.org/10.1016/j.amepre.2016.08.010.

37 Ioannidis, JPA, Stuart, ME, Brownlee, S, and Strite, SA 2017, 'How to Survive the Medical Misinformation Mess', *European Journal of Clinical Investigation*, vol 47, no 11, pp 795–802, doi.org/10.1111/eci.12834.

38 Bero, L 2019, 'When Big Companies Fund Academic Research, the Truth Often Comes Last', *The Conversation*, viewed 18 December 2024, https://theconversation.com/when-big-companies-fund-academic-research-the-truth-often-comes-last-119164.

39 Suzuki, M, Webb, D, and Small, R 2022, 'Competing Frames in Global Health Governance: An Analysis of Stakeholder Influence on the Political Declaration on Non-Communicable Diseases', *International Journal of Health Policy and Management*, vol 11, no 7, pp 1078–1089, doi.org/10.34172/ijhpm.2020.257.

40 Costello, S, Cockburn, M, Bronstein, J, Zhang, X, and Ritz, B 2009, 'Parkinson's Disease and Residential Exposure to Maneb and Paraquat from Agricultural Applications in the Central Valley of California', *American Journal of Epidemiology*, vol 169, no 8, pp 919–926, doi.

org/10.1093/aje/kwp006.

41 European Parliament 2023, 'Culling of Cows and Restriction of Livestock Farming in the EU', viewed 20 January 2025, https://www.europarl. europa.eu/doceo/document/E-9-2023-002312_EN.html.

42 Casselberry, I 2024, 'Paris Olympics 2024: Food Becoming an Issue for Athletes in Olympic Village', *Yahoo! Sports*, viewed 18 December 2024, https://sports.yahoo.com/paris-olympics-2024-food-becoming-an-issue-for-athletes-in-olympic-village-192803761.html.

43 C40 Cities n.d., *C40 Cities – A Global Network of Mayors Taking Urgent Climate Action*, viewed 18 December 2024, https://www.c40.org/.

44 Higgs, K 2021, 'How the World Embraced Consumerism', *BBC*, viewed 18 December 2024, https://www.bbc.com/future/article/20210120-how-the-world-became-consumerist.

Chapter 7

1 Australian Institute of Health and Welfare 2024, 'Overweight and Obesity', *Australian Government*, viewed 12 December 2024, https://www.aihw.gov.au/reports/overweight-obesity/overweight-and-obesity/contents/summary.

2 Heart Foundation 2024, 'Key Statistics: Risk Factors for Cardiovascular Disease', viewed 13 December 2024, https://www.heartfoundation.org.au/your-heart/evidence-and-statistics/key-statistics-risk-factors-for-heart-disease.

3 Carey, RM, Muntner, P, Bosworth, HB, and Whelton, PK 2018, 'Prevention and Control of Hypertension: JACC Health Promotion Series', *Journal of the American College of Cardiology*, vol 72, no 11, pp 1278–1293, doi.org/10.1016/j.jacc.2018.07.008.

4 Healthdirect 2022, 'Pre-Diabetes', *Australian Government*, viewed 16 December 2024, https://www.healthdirect.gov.au/pre-diabetes; Diabetes Australia n.d., 'Pre-Diabetes', viewed 16 December 2024, https://www.diabetesaustralia.com.au/about-diabetes/pre-diabetes/.

5 Mishra, A, Podder, V, Modgil, S, Khosla, R, Anand, A, Nagarathna, R, Malhotra, R, and Nagendra, HR 2020, 'Higher Perceived Stress and Poor Glycemic Changes in Prediabetics and Diabetics Among Indian Population', *Journal of Medicine and Life*, vol 13, no 2, pp 132–137, doi.org/10.25122/jml-2019-0055.

6 Australian Institute of Health and Welfare 2024, 'Diabetes: Australian

Facts', *Australian Government,* viewed 16 December 2024, https://www.aihw.gov.au/reports/diabetes/diabetes/contents/how-common-is-diabetes/gestational-diabetes.

7   Rodolaki, K, Pergialiotis, V, Iakovidou, N, Boutsikou, T, Iliodromiti, Z, and Kanaka-Gantenbein, C 2023, 'The Impact of Maternal Diabetes on the Future Health and Neurodevelopment of the Offspring: A Review of the Evidence', *Frontiers in Endocrinology,* vol 14, doi.org/10.3389/fendo.2023.1125628.

8   Nichols, L 2015, *Real Food for Gestational Diabetes: An Effective Alternative to the Conventional Nutrition Approach,* Lily Nichols.

9   Boyle, J and Teede, H 2012, 'Polycystic Ovary Syndrome and Update', *Australian Family Physician,* vol 41, no 10, https://www.racgp.org.au/afp/2012/october/polycystic-ovary-syndrome.

10   Smith, IAR, McLeod, N, and Rashid, P 2010, 'Erectile Dysfunction – When Tablets Don't Work', *Australian Family Physician,* vol 39, no 5, https://www.racgp.org.au/afp/2010/may/erectile-dysfunction-when-tablets-don-t-work.

11   Teng, ML, Ng, CH, Huang, DQ, Chan, KE, Tan, DJ, Lim, WH, Yang, JD, Tan, E, and Muthiah, MD 2023, 'Global Incidence and Prevalence of Nonalcoholic Fatty Liver Disease', *Clinical and Molecular Hepatology,* vol 29, doi.org/10.3350/cmh.2022.0365.

12   Healthdirect 2023, 'Fatty Liver', viewed 16 December 2024, https://www.healthdirect.gov.au/fatty-liver; University of Western Australia 2017, 'Health of Parents Before and During Pregnancy Linked to Fatty Liver in Teenagers', viewed 16 December 2024, https://www.news.uwa.edu.au/archive/201707129772/international/health-parents-and-during-pregnancy-linked-fatty-liver-teenagers/; SBS News 2017, 'Kids' Poor Diet Linked to Fatty Liver', viewed 16 December 2024, https://www.sbs.com.au/news/article/kids-poor-diet-linked-to-fatty-liver/vb9i2cc5i.

13   Healthdirect 2023, 'Tooth Decay', viewed 16 December 2024, https://www.healthdirect.gov.au/tooth-decay; Department of Health and Aged Care n.d., 'Dental Health', *Australian Government,* viewed 16 December 2024, https://www.health.gov.au/topics/dental-health.

Chapter 8

1   Machado, PP, Steele, EM, Levy, RB, Sui, Z, Rangan, A, Woods, J, Gill, T, Scrinis, G, and Monteiro, C 2019, 'Ultra-Processed Foods and Recommended Intake Levels of Nutrients Linked to Non-Communicable

Diseases in Australia: Evidence from a Nationally Representative Cross-Sectional Study', *BMJ Open*, vol 9, no 8, doi.org/10.1136/bmjopen-2019-029544; Australian Bureau of Statistics 2023, 'Health Conditions Prevalence', viewed 19 December 2024, https://www.abs.gov.au/statistics/health/health-conditions-and-risks/health-conditions-prevalence/latest-release.

2   Layman, DK, Anthony, TG, Rasmussen, BB, Adams, SH, Lynch, CJ, Brinkworth, GD, and Davis, TA 2015, 'Defining Meal Requirements for Protein to Optimize Metabolic Roles of Amino Acids', *American Journal of Clinical Nutrition*, vol 101, no 6, doi.org/10.3945/ajcn.114.084053.

3   Teicholz, N 2023, 'A Short History of Saturated Fat: The Making and Unmaking of a Scientific Consensus', *Current Opinion in Endocrinology, Diabetes, and Obesity*, vol 30, no 1, pp 65–71, doi.org/10.1097/MED.0000000000000791.

4   World Health Organization 2020, 'Healthy Diet', viewed 19 December 2024, https://www.who.int/news-room/fact-sheets/detail/healthy-diet.

5   Harvard Health Publishing 2021, 'Know the Facts about Fat', *Harvard Medical School*, viewed 19 December 2024, https://www.health.harvard.edu/staying-healthy/know-the-facts-about-fats.

6   Eat for Health n.d., 'Macronutrient Balance', *Australian Government*, viewed 19 December 2024, https://www.eatforhealth.gov.au/nutrient-reference-values/chronic-disease/macronutrient-balance.

Chapter 9

1   Teicholz, N 2023, 'Harvard Has Been Anti-Meat for 30+ Years – Why?', *Substack*, viewed 19 December 2024, https://unsettledscience.substack.com/p/harvard-has-been-anti-meat-for-30.

2   International Agency for Research on Cancer 2015, 'IARC Monographs Evaluate Consumption of Red Meat and Processed Meat', *World Health Organization*, viewed 19 December 2024, https://www.iarc.who.int/wp-content/uploads/2018/07/pr240_E.pdf.

3   Wood, AC, Graca, G, Gadgil, M, Senn, MK, Allison, MA, Tzoulaki, I, Greenland, P, Ebbels, T, Elliott, P, Goodarzi, MO, Tracy, R, Rotter, JI, Herrington, D 2023, 'Untargeted Metabolomic Analysis Investigating Links Between Unprocessed Red Meat Intake and Markers of Inflammation', *American Journal of Clinical Nutrition*, vol 118, no 5, pp 989–999, doi.org/10.1016/j.ajcnut.2023.08.018.

4   Meat & Livestock Australia 2024, 'B.CCH.2124 - 2021 Greenhouse

Gas Footprint of the Red Meat Industry', viewed 19 December 2024, https://www.mla.com.au/research-and-development/reports/2026/b.cch.2124---2021-greenhouse-gas-footprint-of-the-red-meat-industry/.

5   Teicholz, N 2023, A Short History of Saturated Fat: The Making and Unmaking of a Scientific Consensus', *Current Opinion in Endocrinology, Diabetes, and Obesity*, vol 30, no 1, pp 65–71. https://doi.org/10.1097/MED.0000000000000791.

6   Vitali, C, Wellington, CL, and Calabresi, L 2014, 'HDL and Cholesterol Handling in the Brain,' *Cardiovascular Research*, vol 103, no 3, pp 405–413, https://doi.org/10.1093/cvr/cvu148.

7   Teicholz, N 2023, 'A Short History of Saturated Fat: The Making and Unmaking of a Scientific Consensus', *Current Opinion in Endocrinology, Diabetes, and Obesity*, vol 30, no 1, pp 65–71, doi.org/10.1097/MED.0000000000000791.

8   Mayo Clinic Press 2024, 'Full-Fat Dairy Foods and Cardiovascular Disease: Is There a Connection?', *Mayo Clinic*, viewed 16 January 2025, https://mcpress.mayoclinic.org/dairy-health/full-fat-dairy-foods-and-cardiovascular-disease-is-there-a-connection/.

9   Yao, Y, Suo, T, Andersson, R, Cao, Y, Wang, C, Lu, J, and Chui, E 2017, 'Dietary Fibre for the Prevention of Recurrent Colorectal Adenomas and Carcinomas', *Cochrane Database of Systematic Reviews*, no 1, doi.org/10.1002/14651858.CD003430.pub2.

10 Gracner, T, Boone, C, and Gertler, PJ 2024, 'Exposure to Sugar Rationing in the First 1000 Days of Life Protected Against Chronic Disease', *Science*, vol 386, no 6725, pp 1043–1048, doi.org/10.1126/science.adn5421.

11 Middha, P, Weinstein, SJ, Männistö, S, Albanes, D, and Mondul, AM 2019, 'β-Carotene Supplementation and Lung Cancer Incidence in the Alpha-Tocopherol, Beta-Carotene Cancer Prevention Study: The Role of Tar and Nicotine', *Nicotine & Tobacco Research*, vol 21, no 8, pp 1045–1050, doi.org/10.1093/ntr/nty115.

12 Mead, E 2019, 'So How Much Caffeine Is in Espresso Coffee?' *Aromas Coffee Roasters*, viewed 19 December 2024, https://aromas.com.au/blog/so-how-much-caffeine-is-in-espresso-coffee/.

13 Food Standards Australia New Zealand n.d., 'Caffeine Powders and High Caffeine Content Foods', viewed 19 December 2024, https://www.food-standards.gov.au/caffeine-powders-and-high-caffeine-content-foods.

Chapter 10

1   Huberman, A 2023, 'Dr. Robert Lustig: How Sugar & Processed Foods
    Impact Your Health', YouTube Video, *YouTube*, viewed 14 January 2025,
    https://youtu.be/n28W4AmvMDE

2   Thompson, PD, Panza, G, Zaleski, A, and Taylor, B 2016, 'Statin-
    Associated Side Effects,' *Journal of the American College of Cardiology*, vol 67,
    no 20, doi.org/10.1016/j.jacc.2016.02.071.

3   Kendrick, M 2021, *The Clot Thickens: The Enduring Mystery of Heart Disease*,
    Columbus Publishing, Wales.

4   Kendrick, M 2021, *The Clot Thickens: The Enduring Mystery of Heart Disease*,
    Columbus Publishing, Wales.

5   Nutrition Coalition 2023, 'Many Studies Will Be Excluded from
    Dietary Guidelines Review, Says Nutrition Coalition', viewed
    14 January 2024, https://www.nutritioncoalition.us/news/
    many-studies-excluded-from-guidelines-review.

6   Teicholz, N 2014, *The Big Fat Surprise: Why Butter, Meat, and Cheese Belong in a
    Healthy Diet*, Scribe, London.

7   Teicholz, N 2023, 'A Short History of Saturated Fat: The Making and
    Unmaking of a Scientific Consensus', *Current Opinion in Endocrinology,
    Diabetes and Obesity*, vol 30, no 1, pp 65–71, doi.org/10.1097/
    MED.0000000000000791.

8   Cahill, GF 1971, 'The Banting Memorial Lecture 1971: Physiology of
    Insulin in Man', *Diabetes*, vol 20, no 12, pp 785–799, doi.org/10.2337/
    diab.20.12.785.

9   Kraft, JR 1975, 'Detection of Diabetes Mellitus *In Situ* (Occult Diabetes)',
    Laboratory Medicine, vol 6, no 2, pp 10–22, doi.org/10.1093/labmed/6.2.10.

10 Schofield, G 2013, 'Joseph Kraft: Why Hyperinsulinemia Matters', *GS
    Health and Performance*, viewed 20 January 2025, https://profgrantschofield.
    com/2013/08/16/joseph-kraft-why-hyperinsulinemia-matters/.

11 Kraft, JR 2008, *Diabetes Epidemic & You*, Trafford Publishing, Bloomington,
    Indiana.

12 Reaven, GM 1988, 'Banting Lecture 1988: Role of Insulin Resistance in
    Human Disease', *Diabetes*, vol 37, no 12, pp 1595–1607, doi.org/10.2337/
    diab.37.12.1595.

13 Reaven, G 2002, 'Metabolic Syndrome: Pathophysiology and Implications
    for Management of Cardiovascular Disease', *Circulation*, vol 106, no 3, doi.
    org/10.1161/01.CIR.0000019884.36724.D9.

14   Diabetes Australia 2022, 'Nutrition: Nutrition and Eating Well', viewed 15 January 2025, https://www.diabetesaustralia.com.au/wp-content/uploads/220145-Diabetes-Quick-Guides_Nutrition.pdf.

15   Attia, P 2022, 'How Fructose Drives Metabolic Disease | Rick Johnson, M.D.', YouTube video, *YouTube*, viewed 15 January 2025, https://youtu.be/V02z9mqTWzg.

16   Johnson, RJ, Lanaspa, MA, Sanchez-Lozada, LG, Tolan, D, Nakagawa, T, Ishimoto, T, Andres-Hernando, A, Rodriguez-Iturbe, B, and Stenvinkel, P 2023, 'The Fructose Survival Hypothesis for Obesity', *Philosophical Transactions of the Royal Society*, doi.org/10.1098/rstb.2022.0230.

17   McKenzie, AL, Hallberg, SJ, Creighton, BC, Volk, BM, Link, TM, Abner, MK, Glon, RM, McCarter, JP, Volek, JS, and Phinney, SD 2017, 'A Novel Intervention Including Individualized Nutritional Recommendations Reduces Hemoglobin A1c Level, Medication Use, and Weight in Type 2 Diabetes',
JMIR Diabetes, vol 2, no 1, doi.org/10.2196/diabetes.6981.

18   TEDx Talks 2015, Reversing Type 2 Diabetes Starts with Ignoring the Guidelines | Sarah Hallberg | TEDxPurdueU', Youtube video, *YouTube*, viewed 15 January 2025, https://youtu.be/da1vvigy5tQ.

19   McKenzie, AL, Athinarayanan, SJ, Van Tieghem, MR, Volk, BM, Roberts, CGP, Adams, RN, Volek, JS, Phinney, SD, and Hallberg, SJ 2024, '5-Year Effects of a Novel Continuous Remote Care Model with Carbohydrate-Restricted Nutrition Therapy Including Nutritional Ketosis in Type 2 Diabetes: An Extension Study', *Diabetes Research and Clinical Practice*, vol 217, https://www.diabetesresearchclinicalpractice.com/article/S0168-8227(24)00808-8/

20   Unwin, D, Delon, C, Unwin, J, Tobin, S, and Taylor, R 2023, 'What Predicts Drug-Free Type 2 Diabetes Remission? Insights from an 8-Year General Practice Service Evaluation of a Lower Carbohydrate Diet with Weight Loss', *BMJ Nutrition, Prevention & Health*, vol 6, no 1, pp 46–55, doi.org10.1136/bmjnph-2022-000544.

21   Defeat Diabetes n.d., 'Diabetes Australia and Defeat Diabetes to Empower People with Type 2 Diabetes', viewed 15 January 2025, https://www.defeatdiabetes.com.au/resources/low-carb/diabetes-australia-and-defeat-diabetes-announce-partnership/.

Chapter 11

1   Australian Institute of Health and Welfare 2024, 'Diabetes: Australian

Facts', *Australian Government*, viewed 15 January 2025, https://www.aihw.gov.au/reports/diabetes/diabetes/contents/summary.

2 Australian Institute of Health and Welfare 2024, 'Diabetes: Australian Facts', *Australian Government*, viewed 15 January 2025, https://www.aihw.gov.au/reports/diabetes/diabetes/contents/summary; Diabetes Australia n.d., 'Pre-Diabetes', viewed 15 January 2025, https://www.diabetesaustralia.com.au/about-diabetes/pre-diabetes/.

3 Sainsbury, E, Shi, Y, Flack, J, and Colagiuri, S 2018, 'Burden of Diabetes in Australia: It's Time for More Action', *Novo Nordisk*, viewed 15 January 2025, https://www.sydney.edu.au/content/dam/corporate/documents/faculty-of-medicine-and-health/research/centres-institutes-groups/burden-of-diabetes-its-time-for-more-action-report.pdf.

4 Emerging Risk Factors Collaboration 2023, 'Life Expectancy Associated with Different Ages at Diagnosis of Type 2 Diabetes in High-Income Countries: 23 Million Person-Years of Observation', *The Lancet*, vol 11, no 10, pp 731–742, doi.org/10.1016/S2213-8587(23)00223-1.

5 Diabetes Australia n.d., 'Healthy Diet for Diabetes', viewed 15 January 2025, https://www.diabetesaustralia.com.au/living-with-diabetes/healthy-eating/.

6 Standing Committee on Health, Aged Care and Sport 2024, 'The State of Diabetes Mellitus in Australia in 2024', *Parliament of Australia*, viewed 15 January 2025, https://www.aph.gov.au/Parliamentary_Business/Committees/House/Health_Aged_Care_and_Sport/Inquiry_into_Diabetes/Report.

Chapter 12

1 Jureidini, J 2024, 'Why Are So Many Australians Taking Antidepressants?', *The Conversation*, viewed 15 January 2025, https://theconversation.com/why-are-so-many-australians-taking-antidepressants-221857; Brody, DJ and Gu, Q 2020, 'Antidepressant Use Among Adults, United States, 2015–2018', *CDC*, viewed 15 January 2025, https://www.cdc.gov/nchs/products/databriefs/db377.htm; Australian Bureau of Statistics 2018, 'Mental Health', viewed 15 January 2025, https://www.abs.gov.au/statistics/health/mental-health/mental-health/2017-18.

2 Healy, D 1999, *The Antidepressant Era*, Harvard University Press, Cambridge.

3 Palmer, C 2022, *Brain Energy: A Revolutionary Breakthrough in Understanding Mental Health – and Improving Treatment for Anxiety, Depression, OCD, PTSD, and*

More', BenBella Books, Dallas.

4   Ede, G 2024, *Change Your Diet, Change Your Mind: A Powerful Plan to Improve Mood, Overcome Anxiety and Protect Memory for a Lifetime of Optimal Mental Health*, Yellow Kite, London.

5   Watson, R, Sanson-Fisher, R, Bryant, J, and Mansfield, E 2023, 'Dementia Is the Second Most Feared Condition Among Australian Health Service Consumers: Results of a Cross-Sectional Survey', *BMC Public Health*, vol 23, no 876, doi.org/10.1186/s12889-023-15772-y.

6   Heni, M 2024, The Insulin Resistant Brain: Impact on Whole-Body Metabolism and Body Fat Distribution,' *Diabetologia*, vol 67, no 7, pp 1181–1191, doi.org/10.1007/s00125-024-06104-9.

7   CDC 2025, 'Obesity and Cancer', viewed 15 January 2025, https://www.cdc.gov/cancer/risk-factors/obesity.html.

Chapter 13

1   Australian Institute of Health and Welfare 2024, 'Overweight and Obesity', Australian Government, viewed 16 January 2025, https://www.aihw.gov.au/reports/overweight-obesity/overweight-and-obesity/contents/summary.

2   Statista 2025, 'Estimated Average Daily Macronutrient Intake Per Capita in Australia in Financial Year 2023, by Type', viewed 16 January 2025, https://www.statista.com/statistics/1172045/australia-estimated-mean-daily-macronutrient-intake-per-capita-by-type.

3   Australian Institute of Health and Welfare 2024, 'Overweight and Obesity', *Australian Government*, viewed 16 January 2025, https://www.aihw.gov.au/reports/overweight-obesity/overweight-and-obesity/contents/summary.

4   Australian Bureau of Statistics 2023, 'Waist Circumference and BMI', viewed 16 January 2024, https://www.abs.gov.au/statistics/health/health-conditions-and-risks/waist-circumference-and-bmi/latest-release.

5   Mohan, J, Shams, P, Bhatti, K, and Zeltser, R 2024, 'Coronary Artery Calcification,' *StatPearls*, https://www.ncbi.nlm.nih.gov/books/NBK519037/.